EVIDENCE-BASED PSYCHIATRY FOR PRIMARY CARE PROVIDERS

EVIDENCE-BASED PSYCHIATRY
FOR PRIMARY CARE PROVIDERS

Copyright © 2024 by Huynh Wynn Tran

Cover: Artist Dinh Khai - Book designer: Tien Minh Nguyen

United Buddhist Publisher (UBF)

First printed in California, USA, October 2024

ISBN-13: 979-8-3304-8330-3

© All rights reserved. No part of this book may be reproduced by any means without prior written permission.

HUYNH WYNN TRAN, MD, FACP, FACR

EVIDENCE-BASED PSYCHIATRY

FOR PRIMARY CARE PROVIDERS

UBP UNITED BUDDHIST PUBLISHER

Preface

*In recent years, the United States has faced a significant shortage of mental health specialists, including psychiatrists and psychologists. This shortage has created a gap in care for many patients struggling with mental health conditions, leaving **primary care providers (PCPs)** and **advanced practitioners**, such as **Advanced Pharmacist Practitioners (APPs)**, at the forefront of managing psychiatric care.*

*Primary care providers are uniquely positioned to offer **early intervention**, **diagnosis**, and **ongoing management** of psychiatric conditions, often serving as the first point of contact for patients experiencing mental health concerns. With the right tools and knowledge, they can play a pivotal role in improving mental health outcomes, particularly in underserved areas where access to specialized mental health services is limited.*

Key features of this book include:

- ***Basic Psychiatry Knowledge**: The book provides an overview of common psychiatric conditions seen in primary care, including **mood disorders**, **anxiety disorders**, **psychotic disorders**, and **substance use disorders**. Clear diagnostic criteria, assessment tools, and treatment guidelines are offered to help providers make informed clinical decisions.*
- ***Case Studies and Practical Applications**: Throughout the book, you will find **real-world case studies** that illustrate how primary care providers can identify, diagnose, and treat psychiatric conditions.*
- ***Cultural Competency**: In today's diverse society, culturally competent care is essential for addressing mental health disparities. This book includes specific sections on how to provide **culturally sensitive mental health care** to patients from various backgrounds. It offers insights into cultural perceptions of mental health, barriers to treatment, and culturally specific expressions of distress.*
- ***Pharmacotherapy and the Role of APPs**: Advanced Pharmacist Practitioners are increasingly playing a key role in managing psychiatric conditions, particularly in collaborative care models. This book explores how APPs can contribute to mental health care through **medication management**, monitoring for **adverse effects**, and offering patient education on psychotropic medications. The book highlights the importance of **interprofessional collaboration** and the unique perspective that APPs bring to psychiatric care.*

We hope this book empowers you to provide comprehensive, evidence-based psychiatric care to your patients, enhancing both their mental health outcomes and their overall well-being.

Huynh Wynn Tran, MD, FACP, FACR
Associate Professor of Medicine and Pharmacy
CEO/Founder of Wynn Medical Center Clinics
Los Angeles, California, USA

CONTENTS

Preface	**5**
Chapter 1: Introduction to Psychiatric Disorders and Evidence Based Psychiatry	**15**
1.1. Overview of psychiatric disorders	15
1.2 Roles of primary care provider in mental health	16
1.3. Scope of practice and responsibilities of PCP in managing psychiatric disorders	17
1.4. Evidence Based Psychiatry	18
Chapter 2: Neurobiology of Psychiatric Disorders	**21**
2.1. Understanding the Neurobiology of Mental Illness	21
2.2. Neurotransmitter Systems and Their Role in Psychiatric Disorders	21
2.3. Neuroimaging Techniques in Psychiatric Research	22
Chapter 3: Diagnostic Classification of Psychiatric Disorders	**25**
3.1. DSM-5 Criteria for Psychiatric Disorders	25
3.2. Clinical Assessment and Differential Diagnosis of Mental Disorders	26
3.3. Screening Tools and Diagnostic Tests in Psychiatric Evaluation	26
3.4. Advanced Diagnostic Tools in Psychiatry:	27
Chapter 4: Major Depressive Disorder	**29**
4.1. Overview of Major Depression Disorder	29
4.1.1. Genetic Factors	29
4.1.2. Neurobiological Factors	30
4.1.3. Environmental and Psychosocial Factors	31
4.1.4. Natural Products for Depression	31
4.2. Clinical Presentation and Diagnostic Criteria of MDD	32
4.3. Pharmacotherapy Options: Antidepressants, Augmentation Strategies, and Novel Treatments	35
4.3.1. Antidepressants:	35
A. Selective Serotonin Reuptake Inhibitors (SSRIs)	35
B. Serotonin-Norepinephrine Reuptake Inhibitors (SNRIs)	36
C. Tricyclic Antidepressants (TCAs)	37
D. Monoamine Oxidase Inhibitors (MAOIs)	38
4.3.2. Augmentation Strategies:	39
A. Atypical Antipsychotics	39
B. Mood Stabilizers	40
C. Thyroid Hormone Augmentation (Liothyronine, T3)	42
4.3.3. Novel Treatments:	42
A. Ketamine (IV) and Esketamine (Nasal Spray)	43
B. Psychedelics (e.g., Psilocybin)	44
4.4. Non-Pharmacological Interventions and Adjunctive Therapies	45
4.4.1. Psychotherapy	46

4.4.2. Electroconvulsive Therapy (ECT)	47
4.4.3. Transcranial Magnetic Stimulation (TMS)	47
4.4.4. Vagus Nerve Stimulation (VNS)	48
4.4.5. Lifestyle and Complementary Interventions	48
4.5. ICD-10 for MDD	49
Chapter 5: Bipolar Disorder	**51**
5.1. Overview of Bipolar Disorder Types and Diagnostic Criteria	51
5.1.1. Bipolar I Disorder:	51
5.1.2. Bipolar II Disorder:	51
5.1.3. Cyclothymic Disorder:	52
5.1.4. Other Specified and Unspecified Bipolar Disorders:	52
5.2. Pharmacotherapy Treatment for Acute Manic, Depressive, and Mixed Episodes	52
5.2.1. Acute Manic Episodes	52
5.2.2. Acute Depressive Episodes in Bipolar Disorder	56
5.2.3. Mixed Episodes:	59
5.3. Maintenance Treatment Strategies	59
5.4. ICD-10 for Bipolar Disorder	61
Chapter 6: Anxiety Disorders	**63**
6.1. Overview of Generalized Anxiety Disorder	63
6.1.1. Generalized Anxiety Disorder (GAD):	63
6.1.2. Panic Disorder:	63
6.1.3. Social Anxiety Disorder (SAD):	63
6.1.4. Specific Phobias:	64
6.2. Pharmacotherapy Options: Anxiolytics, Antidepressants, and Buspirone	64
6.2.1. Anxiolytics (Benzodiazepines):	64
6.2.2. Antidepressants:	64
6.2.3. Buspirone:	65
6.3. Psychotherapy and Cognitive-Behavioral Interventions	65
6.3.1. Cognitive-Behavioral Therapy (CBT):	65
6.3.2. Acceptance and Commitment Therapy (ACT):	65
6.3.3. Mindfulness-Based Stress Reduction (MBSR):	65
6.4. Patient Education and Counseling for Anxiety Management	65
6.4.1. Medication Adherence and Expectations:	66
6.4.2. Stress Management Techniques:	66
6.4.3. Sleep Hygiene:	66
6.4.4. Avoidance of Stimulants:	66
6.4.5. Support Systems for General Anxiety Disorders:	66
6.5. ICD-10 for Anxiety Disorders	67
Chapter 7: Schizophrenia and Other Psychotic Disorders	**69**
7.1. Understanding the Psychotic Spectrum	69
7.1.1. Schizophrenia:	69

  7.1.2. Schizoaffective Disorder: 69
  7.1.3. Brief Psychotic Disorder: 69
  7.1.4. Delusional Disorder: 69
  7.1.5. Substance-Induced Psychotic Disorder: 70
 7.2. Antipsychotic Medications: First-Generation vs. Second-Generation Agents   70
  7.2.1. First-Generation Antipsychotics (FGAs):   70
  7.2.2. Second-Generation Antipsychotics (SGAs):   70
 7.3. Adverse Effects of Medications and Monitoring Considerations   71
  7.3.1. Extrapyramidal Side Effects (EPS):   71
  7.3.2. Metabolic Side Effects: 71
  7.3.3. Cardiovascular Risks: 71
  7.3.4. Agranulocytosis: 71
 7.4. Pharmacological and Non-Pharmacological Approaches to Managing Psychosis   71
  7.4.1. Pharmacological Approaches: 72
  7.4.2. Non-Pharmacological Approaches: 72
 7.5. ICD-10 for Schizophrenia and Related Psychotic Disorders   72

Chapter 8: Attention-Deficit/Hyperactivity Disorder (ADHD)   **75**
 8.1. Overview of ADHD and Diagnostic Criteria   75
 8.2. DSM-5 Diagnostic Criteria for ADHD: 75
 8.3. Pharmacotherapy Options: Stimulants, Non-Stimulants, and Alpha-2 Agonists   76
  8.3.1. Stimulants: 76
  8.3.2. Non-Stimulants: 76
  8.3.3. Alpha-2 Agonists: 77
 8.4. Patient Education on Medication Adherence and Lifestyle Modifications   77
  8.4.1. Medication Adherence: 77
  8.4.2. Lifestyle Modifications: 77
 8.5. Collaborative Care with Other Healthcare Providers in Managing ADHD   78
  8.5.1. Role of Psychologists and Behavioral Therapists: 78
  8.5.2. Coordination with Schools and Educators: 78
  8.5.3. Involvement of Pediatricians and Primary Care Providers: 78
 8.6. ICD-10 for ADHD   79

Chapter 9: Substance Use Disorders   **81**
 9.1. Overview of Substance Use Disorders and Addiction   81
  9.1.1. Definition and Diagnostic Criteria: 81
  9.1.2. The Neurobiology of Addiction: 81
  9.1.3. The Continuum of Substance Use: 82
 9.2 Pharmacotherapy Options for Alcohol, Opioid, Nicotine, and Stimulant Use Disorders   82
  9.2.1. Alcohol Use Disorder: 82
  9.2.2. Opioid Use Disorder: 82
  9.2.3. Nicotine Use Disorder: 82
  9.2.4. Stimulant Use Disorder (Cocaine, Amphetamines):   83

9.3. Harm Reduction Strategies and Medication-Assisted Treatment 83
    9.3.1. Harm Reduction Strategies: 83
    9.3.2. Medication-Assisted Treatment (MAT): 83
9.4. Addressing Stigma and Promoting Recovery in Substance Use Disorder Management 84
    9.4.1. Addressing Stigma: 84
    9.4.2. Promoting Recovery: 84
9.5. ICD-10 for Substance Use Disorders 85

Chapter 10: Eating Disorders **89**
10.1. Overview of Anorexia Nervosa, Bulimia Nervosa, and Binge-Eating Disorder 89
    10.1.1. Anorexia Nervosa (AN): 89
    10.1.2. Bulimia Nervosa (BN): 89
    10.1.3. Binge-Eating Disorder (BED): 90
10.2. Treatment: Pharmacotherapy Options and Nutritional Interventions 90
    10.2.1. Pharmacotherapy: 90
    10.2.2. Nutritional Interventions: 92
10.3. Interdisciplinary Approach to Treating Eating Disorders 93
10.4. Supportive Care and Long-Term Management Strategies 95
    10.4.1. Supportive Care: 95
    10.4.2. Long-Term Management and Relapse Prevention: 95
10.5. ICD-10 for eating disorders 96

Chapter 11: Sleep-Wake Disorders **99**
11.1. Overview of Sleep-Wake Disorders 99
    11.1.1. Insomnia Disorder 99
    11.1.2. Hypersomnolence Disorder (Hypersomnia) 100
    11.1.3. Circadian Rhythm Sleep-Wake Disorders 100
    11.1.4. Obstructive Sleep Apnea Hypopnea 101
    11.1.5. Parasomnias 102
    11.1.6. Restless Legs Syndrome (RLS) 102
    11.1.7. Narcolepsy 103
11.2. Pharmacotherapy Options: Sedative-Hypnotics, Melatonin Agonists, and Orexin Receptor Antagonists 104
    11.2.1. Sedative-Hypnotics 104
    11.2.2. Melatonin Agonists 105
    11.2.3. Orexin Receptor Antagonists 105
11.3. Behavioral Interventions and Sleep Hygiene Recommendations 106
    11.3.1. Cognitive Behavioral Therapy for Insomnia (CBT-I): 106
    11.3.2. Sleep Hygiene: 106
11.4. Monitoring and Optimizing Pharmacotherapy for Sleep Disorders 107
    11.4.1. Monitoring Efficacy and Side Effects 107
    11.4.2. Addressing Long-Term Use and Tapering 108

11.4.3. Combination of Pharmacotherapy and Behavioral Interventions	109
11.5. ICD-10 for Sleep-wake Disorders	109

Chapter 12: Personality Disorders — 113

12.1. Understanding Personality Disorders and Diagnostic Criteria	113
12.1.1. Cluster A: Odd or Eccentric Disorders	113
12.2.2. Cluster B: Dramatic, Emotional, or Erratic Disorders	115
12.1.3. Cluster C: Anxious or Fearful Disorders	117
12.2. Treatment: Pharmacotherapy and Psychotherapy in Managing Personality Disorders	119
12.2.1. Pharmacotherapy for Personality Disorders	119
12.2.2. Psychotherapy for Personality Disorders	122
12.3. Collaborative Care Models and Role of Pharmacist Practitioners in Supporting Individuals with Personality Disorders	123
12.3.1. Collaborative Care Models:	123
12.3.2. Role of Advanced Pharmacist Practitioners:	124
12.4. ICD-10 for Personality Disorders	125

Chapter 13: Geriatric Psychiatry — 127

13.1. Special Considerations in Managing Psychiatric Disorders in Older Adults	127
13.1.1. Aging and Mental Health	127
13.1.2. Depression and Anxiety in Older Adults	128
13.1.3. Psychotic Disorders and Delirium	129
13.2. Treatment Challenges and Considerations in Geriatric Psychiatry	129
13.2.1. Age-Related Physiological Changes:	129
13.2.2. Increased Sensitivity to Medications:	130
13.3. Medication Management Strategies to Optimize Safety and Efficacy	130
13.3.1. Start Low, Go Slow	130
13.3.2. Regular Monitoring and Deprescribing	131
13.3.3. Individualized Treatment and Polypharmacy Management	132
13.4. Non-Pharmacological Interventions and Psychotherapy	133
13.5. Caregiver Involvement and Education	133
13.6. Addressing Polypharmacy and Drug Interactions in Older Adults with Psychiatric Disorders	133
13.6.1. Polypharmacy:	134
13.6.2. Managing Drug Interactions:	134

Chapter 14: Pediatric Psychiatry — 137

14.1. Common Psychiatric Disorders in Children and Adolescents	137
14.1.1. Attention-Deficit/Hyperactivity Disorder (ADHD)	137
14.1.2. Anxiety Disorders	138
14.1.3. Depressive Disorders	139
14.1.4. Autism Spectrum Disorder (ASD)	139
14.1.5. Oppositional Defiant Disorder (ODD) and Conduct Disorder	140
14.2. Pharmacotherapy Considerations and Evidence-Based Treatments in Pediatric Psychiatry	140

- 14.2.1. Attention-Deficit/Hyperactivity Disorder (ADHD) — 140
- 14.2.2. Anxiety and Depression — 141
- 14.2.3. Autism Spectrum Disorder (ASD) — 142
- 14.2.4. Oppositional Defiant Disorder (ODD) and Conduct Disorder — 143
- 14.3. Monitoring for Adverse Effects and Optimizing Medication Regimens in Pediatric Patients — 144
  - 14.3.1. Monitoring for Adverse Effects — 144
  - 14.3.2. Optimizing Medication Regimens — 146
- 14.4. Role of Advanced Pharmacist Practitioners in Pediatric Mental Health Care — 147
  - 14.4.1. Medication Counseling: — 147
  - 14.4.2. Monitoring and Management of Adverse Effects: — 147
  - 14.4.3. Collaborative Care: — 147
  - 14.4.4. Addressing Polypharmacy: — 147

Chapter 15: Cultural Competence and Psychiatric Care — 149
- 15.1. Understanding Cultural Influences on Mental Health Beliefs and Practices — 149
  - 15.1.1. Cultural Perceptions of Mental Health — 149
  - 15.1.2. Culture-Bound Syndromes — 150
  - 15.1.3. Cultural Influences on Treatment Preferences — 151
- 15.2. Providing Culturally Competent Care to Diverse Patient Populations — 152
  - 15.2.1. Cultural Assessment in Psychiatric Evaluation: — 152
  - 15.2.2. Culturally Adapted Psychotherapy: — 152
  - 15.2.3. Cultural Competence Training for Clinicians: — 153
- 15.3. Addressing Health Disparities and Promoting Equity in Psychiatric Care Delivery — 153
  - 15.3.1. Health Disparities in Mental Health Care: — 153
  - 15.3.2. Promoting Equity in Psychiatric Care: — 153
  - 15.3.3. Addressing Social Determinants of Mental Health: — 154

Chapter 16: Collaborative Care and Interprofessional Collaboration — 157
- 16.1. Importance of Collaborative Care Models in Managing Psychiatric Disorders — 157
  - 16.1.1. Definition and Key Components of Collaborative Care: — 157
  - 16.1.2. Benefits of Collaborative Care: — 157
  - 16.1.3. Collaborative Care for Specific Populations: — 158
- 16.2. Role of Advanced Pharmacist Practitioners in Interdisciplinary Mental Health Teams — 158
  - 16.2.1. Pharmacist's Role in Medication Management: — 158
  - 16.2.2. Pharmacist's Role in Patient Education and Adherence: — 158
  - 16.2.3. Collaborative Decision-Making: — 159
- 16.3. Effective Communication and Collaboration with Other Healthcare Providers — 159
  - 16.3.1. Building a Collaborative Culture: — 159
  - 16.3.2. Effective Communication Strategies: — 159
  - 16.3.3. Collaborating with Primary Care Providers: — 159
- 16.4. Case Studies and Practical Examples of Interprofessional Collaboration in Psychiatric Care — 160

- 16.4.1. Bipolar Case Study: Collaborative Management — 160
- 16.4.2. Depression and Anxiety Case Study: Treatment of Adolescent in a School Setting — 161
- 16.4.3. PTSD Case Study: Management of Post-Traumatic Stress Disorder in a Veteran — 161
- 16.4.4. Schizophrenia Case Study: Integrated Care in a Community Mental Health Center — 162
- 16.4.5. Psychiatric Crisis Case Study: Emergency Response — 163

Chapter 17: Ethical and Legal Considerations in Psychiatric Practice — 165
- 17.1. Ethical Principles in Mental Health Care Delivery — 165
  - 17.1.1. Autonomy: — 165
  - 17.1.2. Beneficence and Non-Maleficence: — 165
  - 17.1.3. Justice: — 166
- 17.2. Legal Issues and Regulations Governing Psychiatric Practice — 166
  - 17.2.1. Mental Health Laws and Regulations: — 166
  - 17.2.2. HIPAA and Confidentiality: — 166
  - 17.2.3. Informed Consent in Psychiatric Treatment: — 166
- 17.3. Informed Consent, Confidentiality, and Patient Rights in Psychiatric Treatment — 167
  - 17.3.1. Informed Consent: — 167
  - 17.3.2. Confidentiality: — 167
  - 17.3.3. Patient Rights: — 167
- 17.4. Ethical Dilemmas and Professional Responsibilities of Pharmacist Practitioners — 168
  - 17.4.1. Balancing Autonomy and Safety in Medication Management: — 168
  - 17.4.2. Conflicts of Interest: — 168
  - 17.4.3. Collaborating with Other Healthcare Providers: — 168

Chapter 18: Future Directions in Psychiatric Pharmacotherapy — 171
- 18.1. Emerging Trends and Innovations in Psychiatric Drug Development — 171
  - 18.1.1. Novel Mechanisms of Action in Drug Development: — 171
  - 18.1.2. Pioneering Treatments for Specific Psychiatric Conditions: — 171
- 18.2. Personalized Medicine Approaches in Psychiatric Care — 172
  - 18.2.1. Pharmacogenomics in Psychiatry — 172
  - 18.2.2. Biomarkers and Predictive Analytics — 173
- 18.3. Advancements in Neurotechnology and Digital Therapeutics — 174
  - 18.3.1. Neurostimulation Technologies: — 174
  - 18.3.2. Digital Therapeutics and Mobile Health Technologies: — 175
  - 18.3.3. Virtual Reality (VR) in Psychiatry: — 175
- 18.4. Opportunities for Advanced Pharmacist Practitioners in Advancing Psychiatric Pharmacotherapy — 175
  - 18.4.1. Pharmacogenomic Testing and Personalized Medicine: — 175
  - 18.4.2. Medication Management in Neurostimulation and Digital Therapeutics: — 176
  - 18.4.3. Role in Clinical Trials and Research: — 176

Chapter 19. Appendices — 179

19.1. Appendix 1: Commonly Used Psychiatric Medications – Dosing, Indications, and Adverse Effects ... 179
    19.1.1. Antidepressants ... 179
    19.1.2. Antipsychotics ... 180
    19.1.3. Anxiolytics ... 181
    19.1.4. Mood Stabilizers ... 181
    19.1.5. Stimulants ... 182

19.2. Appendix 2: Clinical Assessment Tools and Screening Instruments for Psychiatric Disorders ... 182
    19.2.1. Depression ... 182
    19.2.2. Anxiety ... 182
    19.2.3. Bipolar Disorder ... 183
    19.2.4. Substance Use Disorders ... 183
    19.2.5. Psychosis ... 183
    19.2.6. Cognitive Impairment ... 183

19.3. Appendix 3: Resources for Patients and Caregivers – Support Groups, Helplines, and Educational Materials ... 183
    19.3.1. National and International Organizations ... 183
    19.3.2. Helplines ... 183
    19.3.3. Support Groups ... 184
    19.3.4. Educational Materials and Online Resources ... 184

Chapter 20. Glossary: A-Z Definitions of key terms and concepts related to psychiatric disorders and pharmacotherapy ... **185**

Chapter 1: Introduction to Psychiatric Disorders and Evidence Based Psychiatry

1.1. Overview of psychiatric disorders

Psychiatric disorders encompass a wide range of mental health conditions that affect mood, thinking, and behavior. Major categories include mood disorders (such as depression and bipolar disorder), anxiety disorders, obsessive-compulsive and related disorders, trauma- and stressor-related disorders (such as PTSD), schizophrenia and other psychotic disorders, eating disorders, personality disorders, and neurodevelopmental disorders (such as ADHD and autism spectrum disorder). These conditions can significantly impact an individual's quality of life and ability to function.

1.1.1. Current Status of Mental Health in the US

In April 2023, mental health in the United States continued to be a significant public health concern, with rising rates of psychiatric disorders across various demographics. The COVID-19 pandemic exacerbated mental health issues due to social isolation, economic stress, and health-related anxieties. Depression, anxiety, and substance use disorders, in particular, have seen significant increases in prevalence. Access to mental health services remains a challenge for many, with barriers including cost, stigma, and a shortage of mental health professionals. There has been a push towards telehealth and digital mental health solutions to improve access.

1.1.2. Future Trends in Mental Health

The future of mental health care in the US is likely to be shaped by several key trends:

- Increased Utilization of Telehealth: The pandemic accelerated the adoption of telehealth, which is expected to continue expanding, providing greater access to care for those in remote or underserved areas.
- Integration of Mental Health in Primary Care: There's a growing recognition of the importance of integrating mental health services with primary care to facilitate early detection and treatment.
- Emphasis on Prevention and Early Intervention: Increasing focus on preventive measures and early intervention for mental health conditions, especially in schools and communities.
- Use of Technology and Data: Advances in technology, including artificial intelligence (AI) and mobile health apps, are expected to play a larger role in diagnosing, monitoring, and treating psychiatric disorders.
- Addressing Mental Health Parity: Efforts to ensure mental health conditions are treated equally to physical health conditions in terms of healthcare access and insurance coverage.

1.1.3. Psychiatric and psychological Providers Availability

The availability of psychiatric providers in the US has been a longstanding issue, with a significant shortage of psychiatrists and other mental health professionals relative to the demand for services. Rural areas, in particular, face severe shortages. This has led to long wait times for appointments and care being provided by non-specialists. Initiatives to address this include expanding the workforce by increasing the number of psychiatric residency slots, incentivizing medical students to pursue psychiatry, and enhancing the roles of nurse practitioners and physician assistants in mental health care. Additionally, the expansion of telepsychiatry services is seen as a critical strategy to mitigate provider shortages.

Overall, while challenges remain in addressing the mental health needs of the population, ongoing efforts aimed at expanding access to care, integrating mental health into broader healthcare systems, and leveraging technology offer hope for improvements in mental health outcomes in the US.

1.2 Roles of primary care provider in mental health

Primary care providers can play a crucial role in psychiatric care, often serving as the first point of contact for individuals experiencing mental health issues. Here are some key roles they play:

Assessment and Diagnosis: Primary care providers are trained to recognize common psychiatric disorders such as depression, anxiety, and substance abuse. They can conduct initial assessments, screenings, and diagnostic evaluations to identify mental health concerns.

Treatment Planning and Management: Primary care providers can develop treatment plans tailored to the individual's needs, which may include medication management, psychotherapy referrals, or lifestyle interventions. They often coordinate care with mental health specialists and other healthcare professionals to ensure comprehensive treatment.

Medication Management: Primary care providers can prescribe and monitor psychiatric medications, such as antidepressants or anxiolytics, for patients with milder or more common mental health conditions. They monitor medication efficacy, side effects, and adherence, making adjustments as needed.

Crisis Intervention and Suicide Prevention: Primary care providers are trained to recognize signs of psychiatric emergencies, including suicidal ideation or acute psychotic episodes. They can provide immediate interventions, such as safety planning, referral to emergency services, or hospitalization when necessary.

Psychoeducation and Counseling: Primary care providers offer psychoeducation to patients and their families about mental health conditions, treatment options, and coping strategies. They may also provide brief counseling or supportive interventions to address stressors and promote resilience.

Collaboration and Referral: Primary care providers collaborate with mental health specialists, such as psychiatrists, psychologists, and social workers, to ensure continuity of care. They make appropriate referrals for specialized assessment and treatment when patients require more intensive or complex psychiatric interventions.

Prevention and Health Promotion: Primary care providers play a role in preventing mental health problems by addressing risk factors, promoting healthy lifestyles, and offering preventive interventions. They may screen for mental health issues during routine health visits and provide early interventions to prevent escalation.

Integrated Care: With the growing recognition of the interconnectedness of physical and mental health, primary care providers increasingly offer integrated care models that address both physical and mental health needs holistically. This approach improves access to mental health services and reduces stigma associated with seeking help from specialized providers.

Overall, primary care providers play a vital role in the early identification, management, and prevention of psychiatric disorders, contributing to better outcomes and overall well-being for their patients.

1.3. Scope of practice and responsibilities of PCP in managing psychiatric disorders

The scope of practice and responsibilities of primary care providers (PCPs) in managing psychiatric disorders can vary depending on factors such as training, experience, and healthcare system regulations.

- **Initial Assessment and Diagnosis:** PCPs are often the first point of contact for individuals experiencing mental health symptoms. They conduct initial assessments to screen for psychiatric disorders, including depression, anxiety, bipolar disorder, and substance use disorders. They gather medical history, perform physical examinations, and administer screening tools to aid in diagnosis.
- **Treatment Planning and Management:** PCPs develop comprehensive treatment plans based on the patient's diagnosis, severity of symptoms, and individual preferences. This may include medication management, psychotherapy referrals, lifestyle modifications, and complementary therapies. They monitor treatment response, adjust medications, and provide ongoing support and guidance to patients.
- **Medication Management:** PCPs prescribe and manage psychiatric medications for patients with common mental health conditions, such as antidepressants, anxiolytics, and mood stabilizers. They monitor medication efficacy, side effects, and interactions with other medications to optimize treatment outcomes. PCPs may collaborate with psychiatrists or pharmacists for complex medication management.
- **Psychoeducation and Counseling:** PCPs offer psychoeducation to patients and their families about psychiatric disorders, treatment options, and self-management strategies.

They provide counseling on coping skills, stress management, and behavior modification techniques to support patients in managing their symptoms effectively. PCPs also address concerns and misconceptions about mental health to reduce stigma and promote awareness.

- **Crisis Intervention and Suicide Prevention:** PCPs are trained to recognize signs of psychiatric emergencies, such as suicidal ideation, self-harm, or acute psychosis. They provide immediate interventions, including safety assessments, crisis counseling, and referral to emergency services or psychiatric facilities as needed. PCPs collaborate with crisis intervention teams and mental health professionals to ensure timely and appropriate care.
- **Collaboration and Referral:** PCPs collaborate with mental health specialists, such as psychiatrists, psychologists, and social workers, to ensure coordinated care for patients with complex or severe psychiatric disorders. They make referrals for specialized assessment, therapy, or psychiatric consultation when necessary, facilitating access to specialized treatment and support services.
- **Prevention and Health Promotion:** PCPs play a role in preventing psychiatric disorders by addressing risk factors, promoting mental wellness, and providing early interventions. They integrate mental health screenings into routine health assessments, offer preventive interventions, and educate patients about healthy lifestyle habits that support mental well-being.
- **Continuity of Care and Follow-up:** PCPs provide ongoing monitoring and follow-up care for patients with psychiatric disorders to assess treatment progress, address concerns, and prevent relapse. They collaborate with patients, families, and other healthcare providers to ensure continuity of care and support throughout the treatment process.

1.4. Evidence Based Psychiatry

Evidence-based psychiatry refers to the practice of integrating the best available scientific evidence with clinical expertise and patient values to make informed decisions about the prevention, assessment, diagnosis, and treatment of mental health disorders.

This approach emphasizes the use of rigorous research methods, including randomized controlled trials, meta-analyses, and systematic reviews, to evaluate the effectiveness and safety of interventions in psychiatry.

- **Pharmacotherapy and Psychotherapy:** Evidence-based psychiatry involves the use of both pharmacotherapy (medications) and psychotherapy (talk therapy) as primary treatment modalities for various psychiatric disorders. Research continues to explore the effectiveness of different medication classes, such as antidepressants, antipsychotics, mood stabilizers, and anxiolytics, as well as various psychotherapeutic approaches, including cognitive-behavioral therapy (CBT), interpersonal therapy (IPT), and dialectical behavior therapy (DBT).

- **Precision Psychiatry:** There is growing interest in precision psychiatry, which aims to tailor treatment approaches based on individual differences in genetics, biomarkers, neuroimaging, and other factors. Advances in personalized medicine hold promise for identifying more targeted interventions and improving treatment outcomes for patients with psychiatric disorders.
- **Digital Health and Telepsychiatry:** The integration of digital health technologies, including smartphone apps, wearable devices, and telepsychiatry platforms, is transforming mental healthcare delivery. These tools offer opportunities for remote monitoring, self-management support, psychoeducation, and teletherapy, increasing access to mental health services and enhancing patient engagement and adherence.
- **Integrated Care Models:** Evidence-based psychiatry promotes the integration of mental health services into primary care settings and other medical specialties. Integrated care models aim to address the complex interplay between physical and mental health conditions, improve care coordination, and enhance patient outcomes by providing holistic, patient-centered care.
- **Cultural Competence and Diversity:** Recognizing the influence of cultural, social, and environmental factors on mental health, evidence-based psychiatry emphasizes the importance of cultural competence and diversity in clinical practice. Clinicians strive to understand the unique perspectives, values, and experiences of diverse populations to provide culturally sensitive and equitable care.
- **Prevention and Early Intervention:** Evidence-based psychiatry emphasizes the importance of prevention and early intervention strategies to reduce the burden of mental illness and promote resilience and well-being across the lifespan. Efforts focus on identifying and addressing risk factors, promoting mental health literacy, implementing school-based interventions, and fostering community resilience.
- **Neurobiological Research:** Advances in neuroimaging, genetics, and neurobiology have provided insights into the underlying mechanisms of psychiatric disorders. Evidence-based psychiatry incorporates findings from neuroscientific research to inform our understanding of disease pathophysiology, identify potential treatment targets, and develop novel interventions.
- **Implementation Science:** Implementation science seeks to bridge the gap between research evidence and clinical practice by studying the best strategies for integrating evidence-based interventions into real-world settings. This includes examining factors that facilitate or hinder the adoption, implementation, and sustainability of evidence-based practices in routine clinical care.

Chapter 2: Neurobiology of Psychiatric Disorders

Understanding the neurobiological mechanisms underlying psychiatric disorders is critical for advancing both diagnosis and treatment strategies. Recent advances in neuroscience have revealed the complex interplay between genetics, neurotransmitter systems, brain circuits, and environmental factors that contribute to mental illness. T

This chapter explores the foundational aspects of the neurobiology of psychiatric disorders, focusing on the roles of neurotransmitter systems and neuroimaging techniques in understanding and managing these conditions.

2.1. Understanding the Neurobiology of Mental Illness

Psychiatric disorders are not simply psychological in origin but have substantial biological underpinnings. The neurobiology of mental illnesses is multifaceted, involving:

1. Genetic Susceptibility: Genetic factors play a significant role in the development of psychiatric disorders. Many psychiatric conditions, including schizophrenia, bipolar disorder, and major depressive disorder, have been linked to specific genetic variants. Twin and family studies suggest heritability estimates for many disorders (e.g., schizophrenia is around 80%) .
2. Epigenetic and Environmental Influences: While genetics provide a predisposition, environmental factors such as stress, trauma, or substance abuse interact with genetic vulnerability through epigenetic modifications (changes in gene expression without altering DNA). These epigenetic changes can affect brain function and contribute to the onset of psychiatric disorders .
3. Brain Circuitry: Psychiatric illnesses are often associated with dysfunctions in specific brain circuits that regulate mood, cognition, and behavior. For example, in depression, the limbic system, particularly the amygdala, hippocampus, and prefrontal cortex, may show abnormal activity, leading to the emotional and cognitive symptoms characteristic of the disorder . Similarly, disorders like schizophrenia involve disruptions in the default mode network (a network active during rest and self-referential thinking), affecting thought processes .

2.2. Neurotransmitter Systems and Their Role in Psychiatric Disorders

Neurotransmitters are chemical messengers that transmit signals between neurons. Dysregulation in neurotransmitter systems is a core feature of many psychiatric disorders. Several key neurotransmitter systems have been identified as being involved in mental health conditions:

1. Dopamine:

The dopamine system is critically involved in reward, motivation, and emotional regulation. Dopamine dysregulation is most famously associated with schizophrenia. The dopamine hypothesis of schizophrenia suggests that excess dopamine activity in certain brain regions (e.g., the mesolimbic pathway) contributes to the positive symptoms of schizophrenia, such as hallucinations and delusions . On the other hand, diminished dopamine function in the prefrontal cortex is linked to negative symptoms, such as apathy and cognitive deficits .

2. Serotonin:

The serotonin system is associated with mood regulation, anxiety, and impulsivity. Serotonin imbalances are implicated in disorders like depression and anxiety disorders. The most common pharmacological treatments for depression, Selective Serotonin Reuptake Inhibitors (SSRIs), work by increasing serotonin availability in the brain. Low serotonin levels have also been linked to obsessive-compulsive disorder (OCD) and panic disorder .

3. Glutamate and GABA:

Glutamate is the primary excitatory neurotransmitter, while GABA (gamma-aminobutyric acid) is the main inhibitory neurotransmitter in the brain. The glutamate hypothesis of schizophrenia suggests that hypofunction of glutamate signaling, particularly through NMDA receptors, may contribute to cognitive deficits and negative symptoms of schizophrenia . Dysregulation of GABA has also been linked to anxiety disorders and bipolar disorder .

4. Norepinephrine:

The norepinephrine system is primarily involved in the body's fight-or-flight response, affecting arousal and stress response. Dysregulation in this system is implicated in anxiety disorders and post-traumatic stress disorder (PTSD). Medications that target norepinephrine, such as SNRIs (serotonin-norepinephrine reuptake inhibitors), are often used to treat both anxiety and depression .

5. Acetylcholine:

Acetylcholine is involved in cognitive processes, including attention and memory. Alterations in acetylcholine signaling are seen in Alzheimer's disease and other dementias. Reduced cholinergic function is associated with memory deficits, while excessive cholinergic activity may contribute to the development of symptoms such as hallucinations .

2.3. Neuroimaging Techniques in Psychiatric Research

Neuroimaging has revolutionized psychiatric research by enabling the visualization of structural and functional abnormalities in the brain associated with psychiatric disorders. Various neuroimaging techniques are used to study mental illness, including:

1. Structural Neuroimaging:

- Magnetic Resonance Imaging (MRI): MRI provides detailed images of brain anatomy, allowing researchers to examine structural abnormalities in psychiatric disorders. For

instance, patients with major depressive disorder often show reduced volume in the hippocampus, which is associated with memory and emotional regulation . Schizophrenia has been associated with enlargement of the brain's ventricles and decreased gray matter .
- Diffusion Tensor Imaging (DTI): DTI is a type of MRI that assesses the integrity of white matter tracts in the brain. White matter abnormalities are implicated in conditions like bipolar disorder and schizophrenia, where communication between brain regions is disrupted .

2. Functional Neuroimaging:

- Functional MRI (fMRI): fMRI measures brain activity by detecting changes in blood flow. This technique is widely used to examine functional connectivity and how different brain regions communicate during specific tasks or at rest. In conditions like depression, hypoactivity in the prefrontal cortex and hyperactivity in the amygdala during emotional tasks have been observed .
- Positron Emission Tomography (PET): PET involves the use of radiolabeled tracers to measure neurotransmitter activity, glucose metabolism, or blood flow in the brain. It has been instrumental in studying the dopamine system in schizophrenia and the serotonin system in depression .
- Electroencephalography (EEG): EEG records electrical activity in the brain and is used to study the neurophysiological mechanisms underlying psychiatric disorders, such as abnormalities in brain waves during sleep in depression or abnormal synchrony in schizophrenia .

3. Emerging Techniques:

- Magnetoencephalography (MEG): MEG measures magnetic fields generated by neuronal activity and provides high temporal resolution. It has been used in the study of epilepsy, autism spectrum disorder, and schizophrenia .
- Transcranial Magnetic Stimulation (TMS): Although primarily used as a therapeutic tool, TMS is also being employed in research to study the functional roles of specific brain regions in psychiatric disorders. TMS has shown promise in treating treatment-resistant depression by stimulating the dorsolateral prefrontal cortex .

The neurobiology of psychiatric disorders is a rapidly evolving field that offers insights into the underlying mechanisms of mental illness. By understanding the role of neurotransmitter systems, brain circuits, and environmental influences, clinicians and researchers can better diagnose, treat, and potentially prevent psychiatric conditions. Neuroimaging techniques have played a crucial role in uncovering the biological underpinnings of psychiatric disorders and continue to advance our understanding of brain function in mental illness.

References:

1. Sullivan, P. F., Daly, M. J., & O'Donovan, M. (2012). Genetic architectures of psychiatric disorders: The emerging picture and its implications. *Nature Reviews Genetics*, 13(8), 537-551.
2. Klengel, T., & Binder, E. B. (2015). Epigenetics of stress-related psychiatric disorders and gene × environment interactions. *Neuron*, 86(6), 1343-1357.
3. Price, J. L., & Drevets, W. C. (2012). Neural circuits underlying the pathophysiology of mood disorders. *Trends in Cognitive Sciences*, 16(1), 61-71.
4. Whitfield-Gabrieli, S., & Ford, J. M. (2012). Default mode network activity and connectivity in psychopathology. *Annual Review of Clinical Psychology*, 8, 49-76.
5. Howes, O. D., & Kapur, S. (2009). The dopamine hypothesis of schizophrenia: Version III—The final common pathway. *Schizophrenia Bulletin*, 35(3), 549-562.
6. Abi-Dargham, A. (2017). Schizophrenia: Overview and dopamine dysfunction. *Journal of Clinical Psychiatry*, 78(1), 7-10.
7. Blier, P., & El Mansari, M. (2013). Serotonin and beyond: Therapeutics for major depression. *Philosophical Transactions of the Royal Society B: Biological Sciences*, 368(1615), 20120536.
8. Coyle, J. T. (2012). NMDA receptor and schizophrenia: A brief history. *Schizophrenia Bulletin*, 38(5), 920-926.
9. McEwen, B. S., & Morrison, J. H. (2013). The brain on stress: Vulnerability and plasticity of the prefrontal cortex over the life course. *Neuron*, 79(1), 16-29.

Chapter 3: Diagnostic Classification of Psychiatric Disorders

Psychiatric disorders are categorized using structured diagnostic criteria to ensure consistency and accuracy in diagnosis and treatment.

In this chapter, we will discuss the Diagnostic and Statistical Manual of Mental Disorders, Fifth Edition (DSM-5) criteria, the importance of clinical assessment and differential diagnosis, and the key screening tools and diagnostic tests used in psychiatric evaluation.

3.1. DSM-5 Criteria for Psychiatric Disorders

The DSM-5, published by the American Psychiatric Association (APA) in 2013, serves as the standard classification of mental disorders used by mental health professionals in the U.S. and internationally. It provides clear definitions and diagnostic criteria for psychiatric conditions, allowing clinicians to categorize symptoms into recognized disorders.

Key updates in DSM-5:

1. **Dimensional Assessment:** The DSM-5 introduced dimensional assessments alongside categorical diagnoses. This means clinicians evaluate the severity of symptoms and their impact on functioning rather than merely confirming the presence of a disorder.
2. **Cultural Formulation:** The DSM-5 emphasizes cultural context in psychiatric diagnoses, ensuring clinicians consider cultural factors in the expression of symptoms and responses to treatment.
3. **Revisions to Disorder Categories:** Several changes were made to the classification of specific disorders. For instance, Autism Spectrum Disorder (ASD) now includes previous conditions like Asperger's syndrome under a single category. Schizophrenia subtypes were removed, focusing instead on symptom severity.
4. **New Disorders:** Several new conditions were added, such as Disruptive Mood Dysregulation Disorder (DMDD), Hoarding Disorder, and Premenstrual Dysphoric Disorder (PMDD).

Advantages of DSM-5:

- Provides a systematic framework for identifying mental disorders.
- Standardizes diagnoses across healthcare settings and research.
- Improves communication among clinicians, researchers, and patients.

Limitations of DSM-5:

- Critics argue that it relies too heavily on the biomedical model and categorical classification of mental disorders, potentially oversimplifying complex conditions.

- Some feel it pathologized normal behaviors or emotions, leading to overdiagnosis and overtreatment.

3.2. Clinical Assessment and Differential Diagnosis of Mental Disorders

A thorough clinical assessment is essential for diagnosing psychiatric disorders, distinguishing between different mental health conditions, and formulating an effective treatment plan. The assessment process generally involves:

1. Clinical Interview: A structured or semi-structured interview where the clinician gathers information about the patient's current symptoms, past psychiatric history, medical history, and family history. Interviews also explore social, occupational, and interpersonal functioning.
2. Mental Status Examination (MSE): A systematic evaluation of the patient's cognitive function, emotional state, thought processes, and behavior. Key components include appearance, mood, thought content, and insight.
3. Collateral Information: Clinicians may collect additional data from family members, caregivers, or medical records to gain a broader understanding of the patient's condition.
4. Psychosocial and Cultural Considerations: A comprehensive assessment will include evaluation of environmental stressors, cultural background, social support, and coping mechanisms, which may impact the development or maintenance of psychiatric symptoms.

Differential Diagnosis

A critical part of psychiatric evaluation is determining whether a patient's symptoms are best explained by one disorder or multiple disorders. Many psychiatric conditions share overlapping symptoms, making differential diagnosis essential. This process involves ruling out alternative explanations for a patient's symptoms, including:

- Medical conditions (e.g., thyroid disorders, neurological diseases)
- Substance use or withdrawal
- Other psychiatric disorders (e.g., distinguishing between depression and bipolar disorder)

Clinical expertise and comprehensive assessment are necessary to avoid misdiagnosis, which can lead to inappropriate treatment. Diagnostic uncertainty can often be reduced by combining clinical judgment with structured screening tools.

3.3. Screening Tools and Diagnostic Tests in Psychiatric Evaluation

In addition to interviews and clinical observation, a variety of screening tools and diagnostic tests are used to support the diagnosis of psychiatric disorders. These tools help clinicians identify specific symptom patterns and monitor treatment progress.

Common Screening Tools:

1. **Patient Health Questionnaire (PHQ-9)**: A widely used screening tool for assessing depression. It measures the severity of depressive symptoms based on the patient's self-report of how frequently they experience symptoms like low mood, fatigue, and changes in appetite or sleep patterns over the past two weeks.
2. Generalized Anxiety Disorder 7-item Scale (GAD-7): A brief tool used to assess the severity of generalized anxiety. It asks about symptoms such as excessive worry, irritability, and restlessness.
3. Mood Disorder Questionnaire (MDQ): Designed to screen for bipolar disorder, this tool identifies periods of abnormally elevated mood, energy, and irritability, as well as the impact of these symptoms on functioning.
4. Mini-Mental State Examination (MMSE): Used to assess cognitive impairment in older adults, this tool evaluates orientation, memory, attention, language, and visuospatial abilities. It is commonly used to screen for dementia or delirium.
5. Alcohol Use Disorders Identification Test (AUDIT): Developed by the World Health Organization (WHO), this tool helps identify harmful alcohol consumption and the risk of alcohol use disorders.

3.4. Advanced Diagnostic Tools in Psychiatry:

In some cases, clinicians may use more sophisticated tools to aid diagnosis or rule out medical causes of psychiatric symptoms:

1. Neuroimaging (e.g., MRI, CT scans): Neuroimaging techniques can help identify structural brain abnormalities that may be associated with psychiatric symptoms (e.g., tumors, traumatic brain injury). These tests are not diagnostic on their own but can provide valuable information when a neurological cause is suspected.
2. Electroencephalography (EEG): EEG can be used to rule out seizure disorders or other neurological conditions that may mimic psychiatric symptoms, such as non-epileptic seizures or delirium.
3. Laboratory Testing: Blood tests may be conducted to check for metabolic or endocrine abnormalities (e.g., thyroid dysfunction, vitamin deficiencies) that could contribute to psychiatric symptoms.
4. Genetic Testing: Although not routinely used in clinical practice, genetic tests may be helpful in specific cases, particularly for early-onset or treatment-resistant psychiatric disorders. Some genetic markers are associated with increased risk for conditions like schizophrenia and bipolar disorder.

The process of diagnosing psychiatric disorders involves the integration of DSM-5 criteria, clinical assessment, differential diagnosis, and the use of screening and diagnostic tools. Combining these elements allows clinicians to create a comprehensive understanding of a patient's mental health and develop effective treatment strategies.

The DSM-5 provides a structured approach to classification, but the use of clinical expertise and individualized assessment remains crucial in accurately diagnosing and managing psychiatric disorders.

References:

1. American Psychiatric Association. (2013). *Diagnostic and Statistical Manual of Mental Disorders* (5th ed.).
2. Spitzer, R. L., Williams, J. B. W., Kroenke, K., et al. (1999). *Patient Health Questionnaire (PHQ-9)*. JAMA.
3. Löwe, B., Decker, O., Müller, S., et al. (2008). *Generalized Anxiety Disorder 7-item Scale (GAD-7)*. Journal of Affective Disorders.
4. World Health Organization (WHO). (2001). *Alcohol Use Disorders Identification Test (AUDIT)*. WHO

Chapter 4: Major Depressive Disorder

> ➤ *Major Depressive Disorder (MDD) is a serious mental condition characterized by persistent feelings of sadness, loss of interest or pleasure, and a range of cognitive and physical symptoms.*
>
> ➤ *It significantly impairs daily functioning and quality of life. MDD may result from a combination of genetic, biological, environmental, and psychosocial factors.*
>
> ➤ *Common treatments include psychotherapy, medications, and lifestyle changes. Early diagnosis and intervention are critical for improving outcomes and reducing the risk of relapse*

Major Depressive Disorder (MDD) is one of the most common and disabling mental health conditions globally. It is characterized by persistent feelings of sadness, loss of interest in previously enjoyable activities, and a range of cognitive and physical symptoms that can significantly impair daily functioning. This chapter will cover the etiology and pathophysiology, clinical presentation and diagnostic criteria, pharmacotherapy options, and non-pharmacological interventions in treating MDD.

4.1. Overview of Major Depression Disorder

The causes of Major Depressive Disorder (MDD) are multifactorial and involve complex interactions between genetic, neurobiological, environmental, and psychosocial factors. Each of these factors contributes in different ways to the risk and development of MDD, influencing how the disorder presents and progresses. Below is an elaboration of the various contributing factors:

4.1.1. Genetic Factors

- **Heritability of MDD:**
  Genetic predisposition plays a substantial role in the risk of developing MDD. Studies have estimated that heritability accounts for approximately 40% of the risk for depression. Family studies have shown that individuals with a **first-degree relative** (such as a parent or sibling) who has MDD are at a significantly higher risk of developing the disorder themselves. Twin studies also support this finding, with higher concordance rates of depression in **identical twins** compared to **fraternal twins**.

- **Genetic Variants:**
  Specific genes associated with neurotransmitter function, particularly those involving **serotonin**, **norepinephrine**, and **dopamine**, have been implicated in depression. One gene that has received considerable attention is the **serotonin transporter gene (5-HTTLPR)**. Variations in this gene are thought to influence the efficiency of serotonin reuptake in the brain, which may affect mood regulation. However, the association

between specific genes and depression is complex, and genetic susceptibility likely interacts with environmental stressors (gene-environment interaction) to trigger depressive episodes.

4.1.2. Neurobiological Factors

Neurotransmitter Dysregulation

- **Monoamine Hypothesis:**
  One of the most well-known theories of depression is the **monoamine hypothesis**, which posits that MDD results from a deficiency in key neurotransmitters, such as **serotonin, norepinephrine**, and **dopamine**. These neurotransmitters are involved in regulating mood, arousal, reward, and stress responses. The idea that low levels of these chemicals contribute to depressive symptoms has driven the development of many antidepressant medications, such as **Selective Serotonin Reuptake Inhibitors (SSRIs)** and **Serotonin-Norepinephrine Reuptake Inhibitors (SNRIs)**. However, this hypothesis alone does not fully explain the complexity of depression, as some individuals do not respond to treatments that target these neurotransmitters.

Hypothalamic-Pituitary-Adrenal (HPA) Axis Dysfunction

- **Stress Response System:**
  The **HPA axis** is the body's central stress response system, regulating the release of **cortisol**, a stress hormone. Dysregulation of the HPA axis is commonly observed in individuals with MDD. Many patients with depression show elevated cortisol levels, particularly in the morning, and an exaggerated stress response. Chronic hyperactivation of the HPA axis can lead to **neurotoxic effects**, contributing to changes in brain structure and function that are associated with depression. This dysfunction is particularly prominent in **severe or treatment-resistant depression**, where patients often exhibit abnormal responses to stress and high levels of anxiety.

Neuroinflammation

- **Role of Inflammation in Depression:**
  Emerging research has highlighted the role of **inflammation** in the pathophysiology of MDD. Elevated levels of **pro-inflammatory cytokines** such as **interleukin-6 (IL-6)** and **tumor necrosis factor-alpha (TNF-α)** have been detected in some individuals with depression. These cytokines can influence brain function, potentially leading to changes in mood, motivation, and cognition. Chronic inflammation may disrupt the balance of neurotransmitters, impair neuroplasticity, and contribute to **neurodegeneration** in areas of the brain implicated in depression, such as the hippocampus. This has led to interest in exploring **anti-inflammatory treatments** as a novel therapeutic avenue for individuals with treatment-resistant depression.

Neuroplasticity and Brain Circuits

- **Reduced Neuroplasticity:**
Neuroplasticity refers to the brain's ability to adapt, reorganize, and form new neural connections. In individuals with MDD, **reduced neuroplasticity** has been observed, particularly in areas like the **prefrontal cortex** (involved in decision-making and emotion regulation), the **hippocampus** (involved in memory), and the **amygdala** (involved in emotional responses). Research has shown that people with depression often have **decreased hippocampal volume**, which is associated with cognitive deficits, particularly in memory and learning. **Hyperactivity in the amygdala** is linked to emotional dysregulation, leading to heightened negative emotions such as fear, sadness, and anxiety.

4.1.3. Environmental and Psychosocial Factors

Chronic Stress and Adverse Life Events

- **Life Stressors as Triggers:**
Environmental stressors such as **chronic stress**, **trauma**, **loss**, or **abuse** are well-established risk factors for the development of MDD. Stressful life events can interact with a genetic predisposition to trigger the onset of depressive episodes. For example, individuals with a history of childhood trauma may be more vulnerable to depression, especially when they encounter additional stressors in adulthood.
- **Gene-Environment Interaction:**
The interplay between genetic predisposition and environmental stressors is crucial in understanding the development of depression. For instance, individuals with certain genetic variants (such as those affecting serotonin transport) may be more sensitive to stress and therefore more likely to develop MDD when exposed to chronic stress or traumatic events.

Psychosocial Factors

- **Social Isolation:**
Social isolation, **lack of social support**, and **financial difficulties** are common psychosocial factors that contribute to the onset and persistence of depression. Social connectedness is protective against depression, while isolation can exacerbate feelings of loneliness, worthlessness, and despair. Individuals who lack supportive relationships or face ongoing social stressors may be at higher risk for depression.
- **Socioeconomic Factors:**
Financial hardship, job insecurity, and poverty can lead to chronic stress, which, in turn, increases the risk of depression. Socioeconomic disadvantage can also limit access to mental health care and social support, contributing to the chronicity of depression.

4.1.4. Natural Products for Depression

While conventional pharmacological treatments for depression remain the cornerstone of treatment, some individuals explore **natural products** as alternatives or adjuncts to traditional therapies. While evidence supporting the effectiveness of these remedies is often limited, they remain popular options.

St. John's Wort

- **Mechanism and Use:**
  St. John's wort is an herbal remedy that has been used as a treatment for mild to moderate depression. It is believed to work by inhibiting the reuptake of serotonin, dopamine, and norepinephrine, similar to some antidepressants.
- **Caution:**
  St. John's wort is a **broad-spectrum inducer of the CYP450 enzyme system**, meaning it can significantly interact with other medications by increasing their metabolism. It can reduce the effectiveness of drugs such as oral contraceptives, anticoagulants, and certain antidepressants. Additionally, when used in combination with other serotonergic medications, it can increase the risk of **serotonin syndrome**.

S-Adenosylmethionine (SAMe)

- **Mechanism and Use:**
  SAMe is a naturally occurring compound involved in the production and metabolism of neurotransmitters such as serotonin, dopamine, and norepinephrine. It has been suggested as an adjunct treatment for depression, particularly in cases where patients prefer not to use prescription medications.
- **Caution:**
  SAMe should be used with caution when combined with other antidepressants due to the risk of serotonin syndrome. More research is needed to establish its safety and efficacy.

Valerian

- **Mechanism and Use:**
  Valerian is typically used as an herbal remedy for insomnia and anxiety, but it may also have mild antidepressant effects due to its role in modulating GABAergic neurotransmission.
- **Caution:**
  Valerian can cause sedation and should not be combined with other CNS depressants (e.g., alcohol, benzodiazepines), as this can lead to excessive drowsiness or impaired cognitive function.

4.2. Clinical Presentation and Diagnostic Criteria of MDD

According to the DSM-5 (Diagnostic and Statistical Manual of Mental Disorders, Fifth Edition), for a diagnosis of MDD, **five or more of the following symptoms** must be present for at least two weeks, with **at least one of the symptoms being either a depressed mood or**

anhedonia. These symptoms must also cause significant distress or impairment in social, occupational, or other important areas of functioning.

1. Depressed Mood

- **Definition:** A persistent feeling of sadness, emptiness, or hopelessness. The individual may feel down most of the day, nearly every day, and this feeling may be reported subjectively (e.g., "feeling sad") or observed by others (e.g., "appears tearful").
- **Impact:** The pervasive low mood affects the individual's outlook on life and may lead to a withdrawal from previously enjoyable activities and relationships.

2. Anhedonia

- **Definition:** Markedly diminished interest or pleasure in almost all activities that were previously enjoyed. Anhedonia can affect activities ranging from hobbies and work to social interactions and relationships.
- **Impact:** This symptom often leads to isolation, as individuals may no longer feel motivated to participate in activities they used to enjoy, contributing to further decline in emotional well-being and relationships.

3. Weight Changes

- **Definition:** Significant weight loss or gain (e.g., a change of more than 5% of body weight in a month) or changes in appetite, either a decrease or increase. Some individuals may experience a marked loss of appetite, while others may engage in overeating as a coping mechanism.
- **Impact:** These changes in weight and appetite can affect physical health, leading to malnutrition, obesity, and associated medical conditions such as diabetes or cardiovascular disease. The changes may also contribute to body image issues and further emotional distress.

4. Sleep Disturbances

- **Definition:** Insomnia (difficulty falling asleep, staying asleep, or waking up too early) or hypersomnia (excessive sleeping). Sleep disturbances are common in MDD and can exacerbate other depressive symptoms.
- **Impact:** Insomnia may lead to irritability, difficulty concentrating, and fatigue, while hypersomnia can contribute to social isolation and reduced productivity. Sleep disturbances also impair the body's natural recovery processes, worsening both mental and physical health.

5. Psychomotor Agitation or Retardation

- **Definition:** Observable restlessness (e.g., pacing, fidgeting) or slowed movements and speech, often noticed by others. Psychomotor agitation reflects internal discomfort or anxiety, whereas retardation indicates lethargy and physical slowing.

- **Impact:** Agitation can lead to heightened tension and anxiety, while retardation can result in an inability to carry out daily activities, making it difficult to perform tasks at work, school, or home. These changes in movement can also be physically exhausting for the individual.

6. Fatigue or Loss of Energy

- **Definition:** Persistent tiredness or exhaustion, even after adequate rest. Individuals may feel drained of energy and may struggle to perform even basic tasks, such as getting out of bed or completing routine daily activities.
- **Impact:** Fatigue can exacerbate feelings of helplessness and contribute to a downward spiral of inactivity, social withdrawal, and declining physical health. This lack of energy often leads to decreased productivity, worsening occupational and social impairment.

7. Feelings of Worthlessness or Excessive Guilt

- **Definition:** Feelings of being worthless or excessive, inappropriate guilt about real or imagined events. These emotions may not be rational or proportionate to the situation, and individuals often ruminate on perceived failures or shortcomings.
- **Impact:** These feelings often erode self-esteem and lead to a negative self-image, further deepening the depressive episode. Excessive guilt can cause individuals to isolate themselves from others and avoid seeking help, exacerbating feelings of helplessness.

8. Difficulty Concentrating, Thinking, or Making Decisions

- **Definition:** A noticeable difficulty with concentration, focus, or making even simple decisions. Individuals may experience "brain fog," with slowed thinking and an inability to process information as efficiently as before.
- **Impact:** Impaired cognitive function can severely affect job performance, academic achievement, and everyday decision-making. It can lead to frustration and a sense of incompetence, contributing further to feelings of worthlessness and guilt.

9. Recurrent Thoughts of Death, Suicidal Ideation, or Suicide Attempt

- **Definition:** Persistent thoughts about death, not just fear of dying but preoccupation with thoughts of death or suicide. This may range from passive suicidal thoughts (e.g., "I wish I were dead") to active planning or attempts.
- **Impact:** Suicidal ideation is one of the most serious symptoms of MDD and requires immediate attention. The risk of suicide is increased, and timely intervention is critical. Individuals may isolate themselves further or express a sense of hopelessness that life is not worth living, making it crucial for caregivers and clinicians to assess risk and provide support.

Additional Diagnostic Criteria

For an MDD diagnosis:

1. **Functional Impairment:** These symptoms must cause clinically significant distress or impairment in social, occupational, or other important areas of functioning. This means that the person's ability to maintain relationships, work, or engage in daily activities is noticeably diminished.
2. **Exclusion Criteria:** The symptoms must not be attributable to the physiological effects of a substance (e.g., drug or alcohol use) or another medical condition, such as hypothyroidism, which can mimic depressive symptoms. It is essential to rule out any medical causes that could explain the presentation of these symptoms.

Variability in Presentation

MDD can present differently in individuals based on age, gender, and other factors:

- **In Children and Adolescents:** Depression may manifest as irritability rather than sadness. Academic decline, behavioral issues, or social withdrawal can also signal depression in younger individuals.
- **In Older Adults:** Depression often presents with more somatic symptoms, such as unexplained aches and pains, fatigue, or memory problems, which can be mistaken for other age-related conditions. Cognitive impairment may also be more pronounced.
- **Gender Differences:** Women are more likely to experience symptoms such as weight changes, fatigue, and feelings of guilt, while men may exhibit irritability, anger, and substance abuse as part of their depressive episode.

4.3. Pharmacotherapy Options: Antidepressants, Augmentation Strategies, and Novel Treatments

Pharmacotherapy is often a first-line treatment for MDD, particularly in moderate to severe cases. The goal of treatment is to reduce the symptoms of depression, restore functioning, and prevent relapse.

4.3.1. Antidepressants:

A. Selective Serotonin Reuptake Inhibitors (SSRIs)

Examples:

- Fluoxetine (Prozac)
- Sertraline (Zoloft)
- Escitalopram (Lexapro)
- Paroxetine (Paxil)
- Citalopram (Celexa)

Mechanism of Action:

SSRIs work by selectively inhibiting the reuptake of serotonin (5-HT) into presynaptic neurons, increasing the availability of serotonin in the synaptic cleft, which enhances mood regulation.

Side Effect Profile:

- **Common Side Effects:**
    - Nausea
    - Diarrhea
    - Sexual dysfunction (e.g., decreased libido, erectile dysfunction, anorgasmia)
    - Insomnia or somnolence
    - Weight gain (more common with long-term use)
    - Dry mouth
    - Headaches
- **Rare but Serious Side Effects:**
    - **Serotonin Syndrome:** A potentially life-threatening condition caused by excessive serotonin levels, characterized by agitation, confusion, fever, sweating, tremors, and seizures.
    - **Increased Suicidal Thoughts:** Especially in younger patients (<25 years), there may be a transient increase in suicidal ideation during the first few weeks of treatment.
    - **Hyponatremia:** Particularly in elderly patients, SSRIs can cause low sodium levels in the blood, leading to confusion, weakness, and, in severe cases, seizures.

Drug Interactions:

- **With Other Antidepressants:** Combining SSRIs with other serotonergic drugs (such as other antidepressants, triptans, or St. John's Wort) can increase the risk of serotonin syndrome.
- **With NSAIDs and Anticoagulants (e.g., warfarin):** SSRIs may increase the risk of gastrointestinal bleeding when combined with NSAIDs or anticoagulants.
- **With MAOIs:** Co-administration can result in severe serotonin syndrome and is contraindicated.
- **With Antiplatelet Agents (e.g., aspirin):** The bleeding risk may increase.

B. Serotonin-Norepinephrine Reuptake Inhibitors (SNRIs)

Examples:

- Venlafaxine (Effexor)
- Duloxetine (Cymbalta)
- Desvenlafaxine (Pristiq)

Mechanism of Action:
SNRIs inhibit the reuptake of both serotonin (5-HT) and norepinephrine (NE), thereby increasing their concentrations in the synaptic cleft and enhancing mood and pain regulation.

Side Effect Profile:

- **Common Side Effects:**
    - Nausea
    - Dizziness
    - Dry mouth
    - Increased sweating
    - Sexual dysfunction
    - Insomnia
- **Noradrenergic-Related Side Effects:**
    - **Elevated Blood Pressure:** Especially with venlafaxine, dose-dependent increases in blood pressure can occur due to norepinephrine reuptake inhibition.
    - **Increased Heart Rate:** Tachycardia is also a concern in some patients.
    - **Constipation:** Due to reduced gastrointestinal motility from norepinephrine effects.
- **Withdrawal Symptoms:** Sudden discontinuation can lead to discontinuation syndrome, characterized by dizziness, headache, flu-like symptoms, and irritability, especially with venlafaxine.

Drug Interactions:

- **With SSRIs and Other Serotonergic Agents:** Increased risk of serotonin syndrome.
- **With MAOIs:** Contraindicated due to the risk of hypertensive crisis or serotonin syndrome.
- **With Alcohol and CNS Depressants:** May increase the sedative effects.
- **Antihypertensives:** SNRIs may reduce the efficacy of antihypertensive medications due to their norepinephrine-raising effects.

C. Tricyclic Antidepressants (TCAs)

Examples:

- Amitriptyline (Elavil)
- Nortriptyline (Pamelor)
- Imipramine (Tofranil)
- Clomipramine (Anafranil)

Mechanism of Action:
TCAs block the reuptake of both serotonin (5-HT) and norepinephrine (NE) but also affect other receptors, including histamine (H1), alpha-adrenergic, and muscarinic receptors, which contribute to their broader side effect profile.

Side Effect Profile:

- **Common Side Effects:**
  - **Anticholinergic Effects:** Dry mouth, constipation, blurred vision, urinary retention, and confusion, especially in elderly patients.
  - **Sedation:** Due to histamine H1 receptor antagonism.
  - **Weight Gain:** Frequently reported with long-term use.
  - **Orthostatic Hypotension:** Dizziness and lightheadedness upon standing, due to alpha-adrenergic blockade.
  - **Sexual Dysfunction:** Including decreased libido and erectile dysfunction.
- **Serious Side Effects:**
  - **Cardiac Toxicity:** TCAs can cause arrhythmias, particularly in overdose situations, due to their quinidine-like effects on cardiac sodium channels. TCAs are associated with a risk of QT prolongation.
  - **Seizures:** Lowering the seizure threshold in some patients.
  - **Risk of Overdose:** TCAs are potentially lethal in overdose due to their effects on the heart and central nervous system.

Drug Interactions:

- **With MAOIs:** Contraindicated due to the risk of hypertensive crisis.
- **With SSRIs/SNRIs:** Risk of serotonin syndrome, especially with clomipramine.
- **With Antihypertensives:** May exaggerate the blood pressure-lowering effects, leading to increased risk of hypotension.
- **With CNS Depressants (e.g., alcohol, benzodiazepines):** Increased sedation and respiratory depression risk.

D. Monoamine Oxidase Inhibitors (MAOIs)

Common Examples:

- Phenelzine (Nardil)
- Tranylcypromine (Parnate)
- Selegiline (Emsam – transdermal patch)

Mechanism of Action:
MAOIs inhibit the activity of monoamine oxidase, an enzyme responsible for breaking down neurotransmitters such as serotonin, norepinephrine, and dopamine. By inhibiting this enzyme, MAOIs increase the levels of these neurotransmitters in the brain.

Side Effect Profile:

- **Common Side Effects:**
  - Orthostatic hypotension
  - Weight gain
  - Insomnia

- Sexual dysfunction
- Peripheral edema
- **Serious Side Effects:**
  - **Hypertensive Crisis:** Ingesting foods rich in tyramine (aged cheese, fermented foods, cured meats) while on MAOIs can lead to hypertensive crises. This occurs due to the inability of the body to break down tyramine, causing a sharp rise in blood pressure.
  - **Serotonin Syndrome:** When combined with serotonergic agents (SSRIs, SNRIs, triptans), MAOIs can precipitate serotonin syndrome.
  - **Drug-Induced Psychosis:** In rare cases, high doses of MAOIs can lead to manic or psychotic episodes.

Drug Interactions:

- **With Tyramine-Containing Foods:** Ingestion of these foods must be avoided due to the risk of hypertensive crises.
- **With SSRIs, SNRIs, and TCAs:** Severe interactions can result in serotonin syndrome or hypertensive crises.
- **With Sympathomimetics (e.g., pseudoephedrine):** Hypertensive episodes due to increased norepinephrine levels.
- **With Anesthetics or Pain Medications (e.g., tramadol, meperidine):** Risk of serotonin syndrome or severe CNS depression.

4.3.2. Augmentation Strategies:

When patients fail to respond adequately to first-line antidepressant treatments, augmentation strategies are often employed to enhance the therapeutic effect. These strategies involve adding another medication, typically from a different class, to improve response rates. Common augmentation agents include **atypical antipsychotics**, **mood stabilizers**, and **thyroid hormones**.

A. Atypical Antipsychotics

Common Examples:

- Aripiprazole (Abilify)
- Quetiapine (Seroquel)
- Olanzapine (Zyprexa)
- Risperidone (Risperdal)

Mechanism of Action:
Atypical antipsychotics work primarily by modulating dopamine (D2) and serotonin (5-HT2A) receptors in the brain. They differ from traditional antipsychotics in their ability to act on both dopamine and serotonin receptors, reducing the risk of some of the motor side effects seen with older antipsychotics.

- **Aripiprazole:** A partial agonist at D2 and 5-HT1A receptors and an antagonist at 5-HT2A receptors. It helps stabilize dopamine and serotonin levels, potentially improving depressive symptoms when combined with antidepressants.
- **Quetiapine and Olanzapine:** These medications block 5-HT2A and D2 receptors but also exhibit antagonism at histamine and alpha-adrenergic receptors, which contributes to their sedative effects.

Side Effect Profile:

- **Common Side Effects:**
    - Weight gain (more pronounced with olanzapine and quetiapine)
    - Sedation and somnolence
    - Metabolic disturbances (increased cholesterol, triglycerides, glucose)
    - Dizziness and orthostatic hypotension
    - Anticholinergic effects (dry mouth, constipation, blurred vision)
- **Serious Side Effects:**
    - **Extrapyramidal Symptoms (EPS):** Including akathisia (restlessness), tremors, and rigidity, although less frequent than with older antipsychotics.
    - **Tardive Dyskinesia:** Involuntary, repetitive movements, especially with long-term use.
    - **Metabolic Syndrome:** Atypical antipsychotics, particularly olanzapine, increase the risk of metabolic syndrome (characterized by weight gain, hyperglycemia, and dyslipidemia), which may lead to diabetes and cardiovascular complications.
    - **Neuroleptic Malignant Syndrome (NMS):** A rare but life-threatening condition characterized by muscle rigidity, fever, and autonomic instability.

Drug Interactions:

- **With Antihypertensives:** Augmentation with atypical antipsychotics, particularly quetiapine, may lead to additive effects, increasing the risk of hypotension.
- **With CNS Depressants (e.g., benzodiazepines, alcohol):** Increased risk of sedation, respiratory depression, and impaired cognitive function.
- **With SSRIs/SNRIs:** Increased risk of serotonin syndrome, particularly with agents that modulate serotonin receptors (e.g., aripiprazole).
- **With Metformin or Insulin:** Quetiapine and olanzapine may decrease the effectiveness of these medications by worsening glucose control, necessitating adjustments in diabetic medications.

B. Mood Stabilizers

Common Examples:

- Lithium
- Valproate (Depakote)

- Lamotrigine (Lamictal)

Mechanism of Action:
Mood stabilizers, particularly lithium, are commonly used to augment antidepressants, especially in patients with bipolar disorder or treatment-resistant depression. Lithium's precise mechanism in depression augmentation is not fully understood but is believed to involve modulation of neurotransmitters (dopamine, glutamate, and serotonin), second-messenger systems, and neuroplasticity.

- **Lithium:** Increases serotonin neurotransmission and inhibits dopamine release, while also promoting neurogenesis and reducing excitotoxicity.

Side Effect Profile:

- **Common Side Effects of Lithium:**
    - Tremors
    - Increased thirst and urination (polydipsia, polyuria)
    - Nausea, vomiting, diarrhea
    - Weight gain
    - Cognitive slowing or "brain fog"
- **Serious Side Effects:**
    - **Lithium Toxicity:** Symptoms include severe nausea, vomiting, confusion, ataxia, and in severe cases, seizures, and coma. This is more common in patients with renal impairment or those taking interacting medications (e.g., NSAIDs, ACE inhibitors).
    - **Hypothyroidism:** Lithium can reduce thyroid hormone levels, leading to hypothyroidism, which may require thyroid hormone supplementation.
    - **Renal Dysfunction:** Chronic lithium use can impair kidney function, necessitating regular monitoring of renal function (BUN, creatinine).

Drug Interactions:

- **With NSAIDs (e.g., ibuprofen, naproxen):** NSAIDs reduce lithium clearance, increasing the risk of toxicity.
- **With Diuretics (e.g., hydrochlorothiazide):** Diuretics can lead to increased lithium reabsorption, raising serum lithium levels and risk of toxicity.
- **With SSRIs/SNRIs:** There is a risk of serotonin syndrome when combined, particularly if serotonergic antidepressants are dosed high or the patient is on multiple serotonergic agents.
- **With Anticonvulsants:** Combining lithium with other mood stabilizers (e.g., valproate or lamotrigine) may increase sedation and cognitive side effects, though this combination can be effective for severe cases.

C. Thyroid Hormone Augmentation (Liothyronine, T3)

Common Examples:

- Liothyronine (Cytomel)
- Levothyroxine (T4, Synthroid) (used less commonly for augmentation)

Mechanism of Action:
Liothyronine (T3) is often used to augment antidepressant therapy in patients with treatment-resistant depression, particularly in those with subclinical hypothyroidism or evidence of low thyroid function. T3 modulates serotonin and norepinephrine pathways and can enhance the therapeutic effect of antidepressants by improving neurotransmitter function and metabolism.

Side Effect Profile:

- **Common Side Effects:**
    - Palpitations
    - Anxiety or jitteriness
    - Sweating
    - Weight loss
    - Tremor
- **Serious Side Effects:**
    - **Cardiac Arrhythmias:** T3 can increase heart rate and lead to tachycardia or atrial fibrillation, particularly in patients with preexisting heart disease.
    - **Osteoporosis:** Long-term use of thyroid hormone can accelerate bone loss, especially in postmenopausal women.
    - **Hyperthyroidism:** Over-supplementation can result in symptoms of hyperthyroidism (insomnia, heat intolerance, weight loss, nervousness).

Drug Interactions:

- **With Anticoagulants (e.g., warfarin):** T3 can increase the effects of anticoagulants, increasing the risk of bleeding.
- **With Beta-Blockers (e.g., propranolol):** Beta-blockers may be used to counteract the side effects of thyroid hormone (e.g., palpitations, tremors), but T3 can reduce the efficacy of beta-blockers by increasing heart rate.
- **With Antidepressants:** Adding T3 to SSRIs or SNRIs may enhance their efficacy, though it may also increase the risk of anxiety and jitteriness in some patients.
- **With Insulin or Oral Hypoglycemic Agents:** T3 can alter glucose metabolism, potentially requiring adjustments in diabetic medications.

4.3.3. Novel Treatments:

For individuals who do not respond to conventional antidepressant therapies, newer augmentation strategies such as **ketamine**, **esketamine**, and **psychedelics** have shown promise. These treatments work through novel mechanisms and have distinct side effect profiles and drug interactions. Below is an in-depth elaboration on the **mechanism of action**, **side effects**, and **drug interactions** associated with ketamine, esketamine, and psychedelics (such as psilocybin) in the treatment of depression.

A. Ketamine (IV) and Esketamine (Nasal Spray)

Mechanism of Action:

- **Ketamine:** A non-competitive N-Methyl-D-Aspartate (NMDA) receptor antagonist that modulates glutamate, the primary excitatory neurotransmitter in the brain. Ketamine blocks NMDA receptors on GABAergic interneurons, leading to increased glutamate release. This cascade activates the brain-derived neurotrophic factor (BDNF) pathway and enhances synaptic plasticity, which is thought to contribute to its rapid antidepressant effects. Unlike traditional antidepressants, ketamine's effects can be observed within hours of administration.
- **Esketamine:** A more potent isomer of ketamine, esketamine also antagonizes the NMDA receptor. It is administered as a nasal spray and is FDA-approved for treatment-resistant depression and depression with suicidal ideation. Esketamine is believed to act similarly to ketamine in enhancing synaptic plasticity and promoting neurogenesis.

Side Effect Profile:

- **Common Side Effects (Ketamine & Esketamine):**
    - **Dissociation:** Feelings of detachment from oneself or the environment (often described as "out of body" experiences).
    - **Nausea and Vomiting:** Common during and after administration.
    - **Sedation and Drowsiness:** Especially in the hours following administration.
    - **Hypertension and Increased Heart Rate:** Due to sympathetic nervous system stimulation.
    - **Dizziness and Headache**
    - **Anxiety or Agitation:** Particularly during the dissociative phase.
    - **Blurred Vision and Sensory Changes**
- **Serious Side Effects:**
    - **Cognitive Impairment:** Long-term use of ketamine may lead to cognitive deficits, including memory and learning issues.
    - **Bladder Toxicity (Ketamine):** Chronic use can cause ketamine-induced cystitis, characterized by urinary frequency, urgency, and bladder pain.
    - **Addiction and Abuse Potential:** Although rare in therapeutic use, ketamine is a known substance of abuse and can be habit-forming in high doses or prolonged use.
    - **Respiratory Depression (rare):** Especially when combined with other sedatives or opioids.

Drug Interactions:

- **With CNS Depressants (e.g., benzodiazepines, opioids):** Co-administration with other central nervous system depressants can increase the risk of sedation, respiratory depression, and hypotension.
- **With MAOIs (Monoamine Oxidase Inhibitors):** There is a theoretical risk of increased blood pressure when used together, though clinical interactions are not well studied.
- **With SSRIs/SNRIs:** No direct contraindication, but ketamine/esketamine's rapid onset of action may affect dosing considerations of other antidepressants.
- **With Antihypertensives:** Ketamine and esketamine can cause acute increases in blood pressure, so caution should be used with patients on antihypertensives, as adjustments may be necessary.

Clinical Use:

- **Ketamine:** Administered intravenously, typically in clinical settings due to the need for monitoring, particularly because of its dissociative and cardiovascular effects. It is used for rapid relief of treatment-resistant depression and acute suicidal ideation.
- **Esketamine:** Administered as a nasal spray in controlled medical environments under supervision, typically for patients with treatment-resistant depression. Patients are observed for at least two hours following administration due to side effects such as dissociation and elevated blood pressure.

B. Psychedelics (e.g., Psilocybin)

Mechanism of Action:

- **Psilocybin:** A prodrug that is metabolized to psilocin in the body, which primarily acts as an agonist at the 5-HT2A serotonin receptor. This activation leads to profound changes in mood, perception, and cognition. Psychedelics such as psilocybin promote neuroplasticity, enhancing the brain's ability to form new neural connections and modify circuits involved in mood regulation. Early research suggests that psychedelics might help "reset" dysfunctional neural circuits related to depression and anxiety.
- **Neuroplasticity:** Psychedelics appear to induce structural changes in the brain, such as increased dendritic growth and synaptogenesis (the formation of new synapses). This may explain their potential long-term antidepressant effects after only a few doses, unlike traditional antidepressants that require continuous dosing.

Side Effect Profile:

- **Common Side Effects (Psilocybin):**
    - **Perceptual Changes:** Visual and auditory hallucinations, altered sense of time and space.
    - **Emotional Lability:** Intense changes in mood, ranging from euphoria to anxiety or fear.
    - **Nausea and Vomiting:** Especially during the initial phases of the psychedelic experience.

- ○ **Increased Sensitivity to Stimuli:** Heightened sensory perception can be overwhelming in non-controlled environments.
- **Serious Side Effects:**
  - ○ **Panic or Anxiety Reactions:** Some individuals may experience acute panic or anxiety during a psychedelic session, particularly if not in a controlled or supportive setting.
  - ○ **Psychosis-like Symptoms:** In rare cases, particularly in those predisposed to psychiatric disorders such as schizophrenia, psychedelics may induce psychotic episodes.
  - ○ **"Bad Trips":** Intense negative emotional experiences during a psychedelic trip, though they are often transient.
  - ○ **HPPD (Hallucinogen Persisting Perception Disorder):** A rare condition where individuals continue to experience visual disturbances (such as flashes of light or halos) long after using psychedelics.

Drug Interactions:

- **With SSRIs/SNRIs:** SSRIs may blunt the effects of psilocybin by downregulating serotonin receptors, potentially reducing its efficacy. This could impact dosage and response in clinical settings.
- **With MAOIs:** Psilocybin is metabolized by monoamine oxidase, so co-administration with MAOIs may increase its potency and duration of action, potentially leading to increased side effects.
- **With Antipsychotics:** These drugs may block the effects of psilocybin, as they often antagonize the 5-HT2A receptor, which is the primary target of psychedelics.
- **With Benzodiazepines:** Benzodiazepines can be used to reduce anxiety or panic reactions during a psychedelic experience but may dampen the therapeutic effects if used preventatively.

Clinical Use:

- **Psilocybin:** Currently under investigation in clinical trials for treatment-resistant depression, end-of-life anxiety, and PTSD. Administration is done in highly controlled settings, often with psychological support to guide patients through the psychedelic experience. Psilocybin sessions are typically accompanied by psychotherapy, with effects lasting for weeks or months after only one or two sessions.

4.4. Non-Pharmacological Interventions and Adjunctive Therapies

In addition to pharmacological interventions, a variety of non-drug treatments play a significant role in managing Major Depressive Disorder (MDD). These therapies are essential components of a holistic approach, especially when tailored to the severity of the depression and individual patient needs. They can be used as standalone treatments in mild cases or in combination with medications for more severe forms of depression.

4.4.1. Psychotherapy

Cognitive Behavioral Therapy (CBT)

- **Mechanism of Action:** CBT is a structured, time-limited therapy that helps individuals identify and modify negative thought patterns (cognitive distortions) and maladaptive behaviors that contribute to depression. The goal is to replace these with more realistic, positive thinking and healthier coping mechanisms.
- **Effectiveness:** CBT is considered one of the most effective forms of psychotherapy for MDD and has been widely studied. It is often recommended as a first-line treatment for mild to moderate depression and can significantly reduce the risk of relapse, particularly when combined with antidepressant medications.
- **Advantages:**
  - Can be equally effective as medication for mild to moderate depression.
  - Focuses on skills that can be maintained over time, reducing relapse rates.
- **Challenges:** CBT requires active participation from the patient, and not all patients may be willing or able to engage fully in the process.

Interpersonal Therapy (IPT)

- **Mechanism of Action:** IPT is based on the idea that depression can be triggered or maintained by difficulties in interpersonal relationships. It focuses on improving communication, resolving conflicts, and navigating life transitions (e.g., loss, role changes).
- **Effectiveness:** IPT has been shown to be particularly effective for individuals whose depression is linked to interpersonal stress or life changes. It is a short-term therapy that typically lasts 12-16 weeks.
- **Advantages:**
  - Effective for patients whose depression stems from relationship conflicts or major life transitions.
  - Helps improve social functioning, which is often impaired in depression.
- **Challenges:** Limited to specific interpersonal issues, which may not address all aspects of a patient's depression.

Mindfulness-Based Cognitive Therapy (MBCT)

- **Mechanism of Action:** MBCT combines mindfulness practices (e.g., meditation, breathing exercises) with cognitive therapy techniques. The goal is to help patients become more aware of their thoughts and feelings and to adopt a non-judgmental stance, reducing the likelihood of being overwhelmed by negative thinking patterns.
- **Effectiveness:** MBCT has been shown to reduce relapse rates in individuals with recurrent depression, particularly in those with residual symptoms. It is especially useful for individuals prone to rumination, a common feature of depression.
- **Advantages:**
  - Enhances self-awareness and emotional regulation.

- o Reduces the risk of relapse, particularly in those with chronic or recurrent depression.
- **Challenges:** Requires commitment to regular mindfulness practice, which may be challenging for some patients.

4.4.2. Electroconvulsive Therapy (ECT)

- **Mechanism of Action:** ECT involves the administration of controlled electrical currents to the brain, inducing a brief, controlled seizure. This treatment alters brain chemistry and can lead to rapid improvement in depressive symptoms.
- **Effectiveness:** ECT is one of the most effective treatments for severe, treatment-resistant depression, particularly in individuals with psychotic features, suicidal ideation, or catatonia. It is typically reserved for cases where other treatments have failed.
- **Advantages:**
  - Highly effective, especially in severe and treatment-resistant depression.
  - Rapid onset of action compared to most antidepressants.
- **Challenges:**
  - **Side Effects:** The most concerning side effect is memory loss, particularly short-term memory impairment. Patients may also experience confusion immediately after treatment.
  - **Stigma:** Despite its effectiveness, ECT remains underutilized due to public misconceptions and concerns about the treatment.
  - Requires anesthesia and multiple sessions, which can be resource-intensive.

4.4.3. Transcranial Magnetic Stimulation (TMS)

- **Mechanism of Action:** TMS is a non-invasive brain stimulation technique that uses magnetic fields to stimulate specific areas of the brain, most commonly the dorsolateral prefrontal cortex, an area implicated in mood regulation.
- **Effectiveness:** TMS has been FDA-approved for treatment-resistant depression and is often used in patients who have not responded to at least one antidepressant medication. It is less invasive than ECT and does not require anesthesia.
- **Advantages:**
  - Non-invasive and does not involve memory impairment.
  - Safe for long-term use and can be performed in an outpatient setting.
- **Challenges:**
  - Requires multiple sessions over several weeks (typically 5 sessions per week for 4-6 weeks).
  - Not all patients respond to TMS, and some may require repeated treatments.

4.4.4. Vagus Nerve Stimulation (VNS)

- **Mechanism of Action:** VNS involves the surgical implantation of a device that delivers electrical impulses to the vagus nerve. The vagus nerve, which connects to the brain, helps modulate mood by influencing brain activity in regions associated with depression.
- **Effectiveness:** VNS is FDA-approved for treatment-resistant depression but is generally reserved for individuals who have not responded to other therapies, including medications and ECT. It can take several months for patients to notice an improvement in symptoms.
- **Advantages:**
  - May provide long-term relief for patients with severe, chronic depression.
  - Can be combined with other treatments like antidepressants or psychotherapy.
- **Challenges:**
  - **Invasive Procedure:** Requires surgery to implant the device.
  - Side effects can include voice changes, difficulty swallowing, and shortness of breath.
  - Requires regular monitoring and adjustments of the device settings.

4.4.5. Lifestyle and Complementary Interventions

Exercise

- Regular physical activity is believed to increase the release of endorphins and other neurotransmitters (e.g., serotonin, norepinephrine), improve sleep, and reduce inflammation, all of which contribute to improved mood and reduced symptoms of depression.
- **Effectiveness:** Numerous studies have demonstrated that regular exercise can be as effective as medication in treating mild to moderate depression. It is also beneficial in preventing relapse and improving overall well-being.
- **Advantages:**
  - Improves both mental and physical health.
  - Has no significant side effects when done appropriately.
- **Challenges:** Motivation can be a barrier for individuals with depression, as fatigue and low energy levels are common symptoms.

Diet

- A diet rich in fruits, vegetables, whole grains, and omega-3 fatty acids may reduce inflammation and oxidative stress, both of which are linked to depression. Emerging research suggests that a Mediterranean-style diet can help improve depressive symptoms.
- **Effectiveness:** While the exact relationship between diet and depression is still under investigation, there is growing evidence that a healthier diet can complement other treatments for depression.
- **Advantages:**

- o Improves overall health and reduces the risk of other chronic diseases.
- o Accessible and non-invasive intervention.
- **Challenges:** Dietary changes require long-term commitment and lifestyle adjustments.

Light Therapy

- Light therapy involves exposure to bright artificial light (usually in the morning) to help regulate circadian rhythms and increase serotonin production. This therapy is particularly useful for individuals with Seasonal Affective Disorder (SAD), a type of depression that occurs during certain seasons (most commonly in winter).
- **Effectiveness:** Light therapy is highly effective for SAD and can also benefit individuals with non-seasonal depression. It typically requires daily exposure to a lightbox for 20-30 minutes.
- **Advantages:**
    - o Non-invasive and easy to use at home.
    - o Provides rapid improvement in mood for individuals with SAD.
- **Challenges:** May cause eye strain, headaches, or agitation in some individuals, particularly if used incorrectly or at the wrong time of day.

Major Depressive Disorder is a complex condition with multifactorial causes, involving genetic, neurobiological, and psychosocial factors. The diagnosis of MDD is based on specific clinical criteria, and treatment often involves a combination of pharmacological and non-pharmacological approaches. Understanding the underlying pathophysiology of MDD has led to advances in both traditional antidepressant therapy and novel treatments such as ketamine and brain stimulation techniques. Holistic care that incorporates lifestyle changes and psychotherapy is essential for improving long-term outcomes in individuals with depression.

4.5. ICD-10 for MDD

The ICD-10 code for Major Depressive Disorder (MDD) is **F32** for a single episode and **F33** for recurrent episodes. Below are the specific subcodes:

- **F32.0**: Major depressive disorder, single episode, mild
- **F32.1**: Major depressive disorder, single episode, moderate
- **F32.2**: Major depressive disorder, single episode, severe without psychotic features
- **F32.3**: Major depressive disorder, single episode, severe with psychotic features
- **F32.4**: Major depressive disorder, single episode, in partial remission
- **F32.5**: Major depressive disorder, single episode, in full remission
- **F33.0**: Major depressive disorder, recurrent, mild
- **F33.1**: Major depressive disorder, recurrent, moderate
- **F33.2**: Major depressive disorder, recurrent, severe without psychotic features
- **F33.3**: Major depressive disorder, recurrent, severe with psychotic features
- **F33.4**: Major depressive disorder, recurrent, in remission

These codes are used to specify the severity and recurrence of MDD in medical documentation.

References:

1. Sullivan, P. F., Neale, M. C., & Kendler, K. S. (2000). Genetic epidemiology of major depression: Review and meta-analysis. *American Journal of Psychiatry*, 157(10), 1552-1562.
2. Malhi, G. S., & Mann, J. J. (2018). Depression. *Lancet*, 392(10161), 2299-2312.
3. Pariante, C. M., & Lightman, S. L. (2008). The HPA axis in major depression: Classical theories and new developments. *Trends in Neurosciences*, 31(9), 464-468.
4. Rush, A. J., Trivedi, M. H., Wisniewski, S. R., et al. (2006). Acute and longer-term outcomes in depressed outpatients requiring one or several treatment steps: A STAR*D report. *American Journal of Psychiatry*, 163(11), 1905-1917.
5. Krystal, J. H., Abdallah, C. G., Sanacora, G., et al. (2019). Ketamine: A paradigm shift for depression research and treatment. *Neuron*, 101(5), 774-778.
6. Cuijpers, P., Karyotaki, E., Weitz, E., et al. (2014). The effects of psychotherapies for major depression in adults on remission, recovery and improvement: A meta-analysis. *Journal of Affective Disorders*, 159, 118-126

Chapter 5: Bipolar Disorder

Bipolar Disorder (BD) is a chronic mood disorder characterized by episodes of **mania**, **hypomania**, and **depression**. These mood fluctuations can significantly impair an individual's ability to function and lead a stable life.

This chapter provides an overview of the **types and diagnostic criteria** of bipolar disorder, explores **pharmacotherapy** for treating acute episodes (manic, depressive, and mixed), and discusses **maintenance treatment strategies** for preventing relapse.

5.1. Overview of Bipolar Disorder Types and Diagnostic Criteria

Bipolar disorder is classified into several types based on the presentation of manic, hypomanic, and depressive episodes. The **DSM-5** provides specific diagnostic criteria for each subtype of bipolar disorder:

5.1.1. Bipolar I Disorder:

- Bipolar I Disorder is characterized by the occurrence of **at least one manic episode**. While major depressive episodes commonly occur, they are not required for the diagnosis. A manic episode is defined as a period of **elevated, expansive, or irritable mood** and **increased activity or energy** lasting at least **one week** (or any duration if hospitalization is necessary), accompanied by three or more of the following symptoms (four if mood is irritable):
    - Inflated self-esteem or grandiosity
    - Decreased need for sleep
    - Increased talkativeness or pressure to keep talking
    - Flight of ideas or racing thoughts
    - Distractibility
    - Increase in goal-directed activity or psychomotor agitation
    - Involvement in risky activities (e.g., unrestrained spending, sexual indiscretions)

A **depressive episode** in bipolar I disorder follows the same criteria as for major depressive disorder (MDD), characterized by a persistent low mood or loss of interest in activities, lasting at least **two weeks**, along with several cognitive and physical symptoms .

5.1.2. Bipolar II Disorder:

- Bipolar II Disorder is characterized by the presence of **at least one hypomanic episode** and **at least one major depressive episode**. Hypomania is similar to mania but is less severe, does not require hospitalization, and does not lead to significant functional

impairment. Hypomanic episodes must last at least **four days** and involve the same symptom criteria as mania, but at a reduced intensity .
- Bipolar II patients tend to spend more time in depressive episodes than in hypomanic states, making depression the primary clinical challenge in this population.

5.1.3. Cyclothymic Disorder:

- Cyclothymic disorder is a milder form of bipolar disorder, involving **numerous periods of hypomanic symptoms** and **depressive symptoms** that do not meet full criteria for a major depressive episode. These symptoms must be present for at least **two years** (one year in children/adolescents), with symptoms occurring at least half the time and no symptom-free periods longer than two months .

5.1.4. Other Specified and Unspecified Bipolar Disorders:

- These categories include individuals who exhibit **bipolar-like symptoms** that do not meet the full criteria for bipolar I, bipolar II, or cyclothymic disorder. For example, individuals with short-duration hypomanic episodes and major depressive episodes may fall into this category.

5.2. Pharmacotherapy Treatment for Acute Manic, Depressive, and Mixed Episodes

Treatment of **bipolar disorder** requires tailored approaches for each type of episode—**manic, depressive, or mixed**—to stabilize mood and address the specific symptomatology. Pharmacotherapy is the mainstay for managing acute episodes.

5.2.1. Acute Manic Episodes

Acute mania is a psychiatric emergency that may require **hospitalization** if the individual poses a danger to themselves or others due to behaviors like aggression, impulsivity, or recklessness. The goal of treatment is to rapidly stabilize mood and control dangerous or disruptive behaviors.

Mood Stabilizers

Mood stabilizers are central to managing bipolar disorder and are often the first-line treatment for acute manic episodes.

Lithium

- **Mechanism of Action:**
  Lithium's exact mechanism is not fully understood, but it is believed to modulate neurotransmitter activity by stabilizing glutamate, dopamine, and serotonin levels. Lithium also inhibits **inositol monophosphatase**, impacting the phosphoinositide pathway, and influences gene expression that regulates neuroplasticity.
- **Side Effects:**

- Common: Tremors, increased thirst (polydipsia), increased urination (polyuria), weight gain, cognitive slowing, nausea, diarrhea.
- Serious: **Lithium toxicity** can cause confusion, ataxia, vomiting, and seizures. Long-term use can lead to kidney dysfunction (nephrogenic diabetes insipidus) and hypothyroidism.
- **Drug Interactions:**
    - **With NSAIDs (e.g., ibuprofen, naproxen):** NSAIDs reduce renal clearance of lithium, increasing the risk of toxicity.
    - **With Diuretics (e.g., thiazides):** Diuretics increase lithium reabsorption in the kidneys, raising serum lithium levels.
    - **With ACE inhibitors and ARBs:** These medications can also decrease lithium clearance, increasing the risk of toxicity.
    - **With SSRIs/SNRIs:** Can increase the risk of serotonin syndrome.

Valproate (Divalproex Sodium)

- **Mechanism of Action:**
  Valproate enhances **GABAergic activity** (an inhibitory neurotransmitter), reduces neuronal firing, and stabilizes mood by inhibiting voltage-gated sodium channels. It also has anti kindling properties, making it effective in rapid cycling and mixed episodes.
- **Side Effects:**
    - Common: Weight gain, tremors, gastrointestinal disturbances (nausea, vomiting), sedation.
    - Serious: **Hepatotoxicity**, pancreatitis, **teratogenicity** (particularly neural tube defects), thrombocytopenia, and polycystic ovarian syndrome (PCOS) in women.
- **Drug Interactions:**
    - **With Antiplatelet agents (e.g., aspirin):** Increases the risk of bleeding due to thrombocytopenia.
    - **With Lamotrigine:** Valproate inhibits the metabolism of lamotrigine, significantly increasing the risk of **Stevens-Johnson syndrome**.
    - **With Warfarin:** Valproate can displace warfarin from protein-binding sites, increasing the risk of bleeding.

Antipsychotics

Atypical (second-generation) antipsychotics are commonly used to treat acute mania, especially when there are **psychotic symptoms** or agitation. These medications modulate both dopamine (D2) and serotonin (5-HT2A) receptors.

Olanzapine

- **Mechanism of Action:**
  Olanzapine blocks dopamine D2 receptors and serotonin 5-HT2A receptors, reducing hyperactivity and stabilizing mood. It also affects histamine and muscarinic receptors, contributing to sedation and weight gain.

- **Side Effects:**
    - Common: Sedation, significant weight gain, hyperglycemia, increased cholesterol, dry mouth, constipation.
    - Serious: **Metabolic syndrome**, increased risk of diabetes, and tardive dyskinesia with long-term use.
- **Drug Interactions:**
    - **With CNS depressants (e.g., alcohol, benzodiazepines):** Increases sedation and risk of respiratory depression.
    - **With Antihypertensives:** May increase the risk of hypotension.
    - **With Carbamazepine:** Carbamazepine induces the metabolism of olanzapine, reducing its efficacy.

Risperidone

- **Mechanism of Action:**
  Risperidone is a potent D2 and 5-HT2A receptor antagonist, reducing dopamine activity in the limbic system to control manic symptoms. It also has some affinity for alpha-adrenergic and histaminergic receptors.
- **Side Effects:**
    - Common: Weight gain, sedation, hyperprolactinemia (which can lead to galactorrhea and menstrual irregularities), orthostatic hypotension.
    - Serious: **Extrapyramidal symptoms (EPS)** at higher doses, tardive dyskinesia, metabolic disturbances.
- **Drug Interactions:**
    - **With SSRIs (e.g., fluoxetine, paroxetine):** These inhibit the metabolism of risperidone, increasing its serum levels and risk of side effects.
    - **With Antihypertensives:** Increases risk of hypotension.
    - **With Carbamazepine:** Reduces risperidone levels by inducing CYP450 enzymes.

Quetiapine

- **Mechanism of Action:**
  Quetiapine blocks both serotonin and dopamine receptors. It also has strong antihistaminergic effects, contributing to its sedative properties.
- **Side Effects:**
    - Common: Sedation, weight gain, dry mouth, orthostatic hypotension.
    - Serious: **Metabolic syndrome**, hyperglycemia, tardive dyskinesia.
- **Drug Interactions:**
    - **With CNS depressants:** Can increase sedation.
    - **With Antihypertensives:** Can lead to additive hypotensive effects.
    - **With Phenytoin and Carbamazepine:** These drugs increase the clearance of quetiapine, reducing its efficacy.

Aripiprazole

- **Mechanism of Action:**
  Aripiprazole acts as a **partial agonist** at dopamine D2 receptors and serotonin 5-HT1A receptors, while antagonizing 5-HT2A receptors. This unique mechanism stabilizes dopamine activity, reducing both mania and psychosis.
- **Side Effects:**
  - Common: Agitation, insomnia, headache, nausea, akathisia (restlessness).
  - Serious: Lower risk of weight gain and metabolic syndrome compared to other antipsychotics, but still possible with long-term use.
- **Drug Interactions:**
  - **With SSRIs (e.g., fluoxetine):** Inhibits metabolism of aripiprazole, increasing its serum levels and risk of side effects.
  - **With CNS depressants:** Increased risk of sedation.
  - **With Carbamazepine:** Reduces aripiprazole levels by inducing CYP450 enzymes.

Benzodiazepines

Benzodiazepines are not mood stabilizers but are used for **short-term management** of agitation and insomnia in acute mania. They are typically used in conjunction with mood stabilizers or antipsychotics.

Lorazepam (Ativan)

- **Mechanism of Action:**
  Lorazepam enhances the activity of **GABA**, an inhibitory neurotransmitter, leading to sedation, anxiolysis, and muscle relaxation.
- **Side Effects:**
  - Common: Sedation, drowsiness, dizziness, cognitive impairment, reduced coordination.
  - Serious: Risk of **dependence**, tolerance, and withdrawal symptoms with long-term use.
- **Drug Interactions:**
  - **With CNS depressants (e.g., opioids, alcohol):** Significantly increases the risk of respiratory depression and sedation.
  - **With Antipsychotics and Mood Stabilizers:** Additive sedative effects may impair cognition and coordination.

Clonazepam (Klonopin)

- **Mechanism of Action:**
  Like lorazepam, clonazepam enhances GABAergic neurotransmission, providing sedative and anxiolytic effects.
- **Side Effects:**

- Common: Sedation, confusion, memory impairment, dizziness.
- Serious: Risk of dependence and withdrawal seizures with long-term use.
- **Drug Interactions:**
  - Same as lorazepam, with increased risk of CNS depression when combined with other sedative agents.

5.2.2. Acute Depressive Episodes in Bipolar Disorder

Treating **acute depressive episodes** in bipolar disorder presents unique challenges due to the risk of triggering **manic or hypomanic episodes**, particularly when using traditional antidepressants. As a result, treatment strategies typically prioritize **mood stabilizers** or **atypical antipsychotics**, which help manage depressive symptoms without the risk of inducing mania. Below is an expanded discussion of the pharmacological treatments used in bipolar depression, including the mechanisms, side effects, and drug interactions of the commonly used medications.

Mood Stabilizers

Lamotrigine

- **Mechanism of Action:** Lamotrigine is primarily a **voltage-gated sodium channel blocker**. By inhibiting sodium channels, it reduces the release of excitatory neurotransmitters like **glutamate** and **aspartate**, which are thought to play a role in mood dysregulation. Lamotrigine is unique among mood stabilizers in that it has more specific efficacy in treating depressive episodes rather than manic episodes, making it a first-line option for bipolar depression.
- **Side Effects:**
  - Common: Headache, dizziness, nausea, blurred vision, fatigue, and rash.
  - Serious: **Stevens-Johnson syndrome (SJS)** and **toxic epidermal necrolysis (TEN)**—rare but life-threatening skin reactions. The risk of SJS is increased when lamotrigine is started at high doses or titrated too quickly.
- **Drug Interactions:**
  - **With Valproate:** Valproate inhibits the metabolism of lamotrigine, significantly increasing its serum levels and the risk of SJS. When co-administered, lamotrigine doses should be reduced.
  - **With Oral Contraceptives:** Estrogen-containing contraceptives can decrease lamotrigine levels, potentially reducing its efficacy.
  - **With Carbamazepine or Phenytoin:** These induce lamotrigine's metabolism, requiring dose adjustments to maintain therapeutic levels.

Lithium

- **Mechanism of Action:** Lithium's mechanism is complex and involves modulating neurotransmitters like **serotonin**, **dopamine**, and **glutamate**. Lithium is effective in

stabilizing mood and reducing the risk of both depressive and manic episodes, although it is often more effective at preventing mania than treating acute depression.
- **Side Effects:**
    - Common: Tremors, weight gain, increased thirst (polydipsia), increased urination (polyuria), gastrointestinal distress (nausea, diarrhea).
    - Serious: **Lithium toxicity**, which can cause confusion, ataxia, seizures, and renal dysfunction. **Hypothyroidism** and **kidney damage** may occur with long-term use.
- **Drug Interactions:**
    - **With NSAIDs (e.g., ibuprofen):** Can reduce lithium clearance, increasing the risk of toxicity.
    - **With Diuretics (e.g., thiazides):** Can increase lithium levels by reducing renal excretion.
    - **With SSRIs or SNRIs:** Increased risk of serotonin syndrome, especially in combination with other serotonergic agents.

Atypical Antipsychotics

Atypical antipsychotics are commonly used to treat **bipolar depression** due to their ability to stabilize mood without inducing mania or hypomania. Two atypical antipsychotics—**quetiapine** and **lurasidone**—are FDA-approved for the treatment of bipolar depression.

Quetiapine

- **Mechanism of Action:** Quetiapine is a **serotonin-dopamine antagonist**, blocking dopamine D2 and serotonin 5-HT2A receptors. It also exhibits strong antihistaminergic and alpha-adrenergic blocking effects, which contribute to its sedative properties. Quetiapine's antidepressant effects are likely related to its activity at the 5-HT1A receptor.
- **Side Effects:**
    - Common: Sedation, weight gain, dry mouth, constipation, dizziness.
    - Serious: **Metabolic syndrome** (increased risk of diabetes, dyslipidemia), tardive dyskinesia, and **orthostatic hypotension**.
- **Drug Interactions:**
    - **With CNS depressants (e.g., benzodiazepines, alcohol):** Can increase sedation and risk of respiratory depression.
    - **With Antihypertensives:** Increases the risk of hypotension.
    - **With Phenytoin or Carbamazepine:** These drugs increase the clearance of quetiapine, reducing its efficacy.

Lurasidone

- **Mechanism of Action:** Lurasidone is a **dopamine D2 receptor antagonist** and a **serotonin 5-HT2A and 5-HT7 receptor antagonist**. It also has partial agonist activity at the 5-HT1A receptor, which may contribute to its antidepressant effects. Lurasidone has

minimal anticholinergic and antihistaminergic activity, making it less sedating than quetiapine.
- **Side Effects:**
    - Common: Nausea, akathisia (restlessness), somnolence, and dizziness.
    - Serious: **Extrapyramidal symptoms (EPS)**, including tremors, muscle stiffness, and tardive dyskinesia. There is also a lower risk of metabolic syndrome compared to other atypical antipsychotics, but it remains a potential concern with long-term use.
- **Drug Interactions:**
    - **With Strong CYP3A4 Inhibitors (e.g., ketoconazole):** These can increase lurasidone levels, necessitating dose adjustments.
    - **With Strong CYP3A4 Inducers (e.g., rifampin, carbamazepine):** These drugs significantly reduce lurasidone levels, making it less effective.

Antidepressants in Bipolar Depression

The use of **antidepressants** in bipolar depression is controversial due to the risk of **manic switch** (i.e., triggering mania or hypomania). When antidepressants are used, they are typically combined with a mood stabilizer or antipsychotic to mitigate this risk. The most commonly used classes are **Selective Serotonin Reuptake Inhibitors (SSRIs) and Serotonin-Norepinephrine Reuptake Inhibitors (SNRIs)**.

SSRIs (Selective Serotonin Reuptake Inhibitors)

- **Examples:** Fluoxetine, sertraline, citalopram, escitalopram.
- **Mechanism of Action:** SSRIs increase serotonin levels in the synaptic cleft by inhibiting its reuptake into presynaptic neurons. This enhanced serotonergic activity helps alleviate depressive symptoms.
- **Side Effects:**
    - Common: Nausea, sexual dysfunction, insomnia, headache, weight gain.
    - Serious: **Serotonin syndrome** (agitation, confusion, tremors, fever) when combined with other serotonergic drugs. There is also the risk of **manic switch** in individuals with bipolar disorder, particularly when SSRIs are used without a mood stabilizer.
- **Drug Interactions:**
    - **With MAOIs (Monoamine Oxidase Inhibitors):** Combining SSRIs with MAOIs is contraindicated due to the risk of severe serotonin syndrome.
    - **With Antiplatelet drugs (e.g., aspirin, clopidogrel):** Increased risk of gastrointestinal bleeding.
    - **With St. John's Wort:** Increases the risk of serotonin syndrome.

SNRIs (Serotonin-Norepinephrine Reuptake Inhibitors)

- **Examples:** Venlafaxine, duloxetine.

- **Mechanism of Action:** SNRIs inhibit the reuptake of both **serotonin** and **norepinephrine**, increasing the availability of these neurotransmitters in the brain. This dual action makes them effective for both mood regulation and alleviating physical symptoms of depression (e.g., pain).
- **Side Effects:**
    - Common: Nausea, dry mouth, increased sweating, dizziness, insomnia, and sexual dysfunction.
    - Serious: **Elevated blood pressure** (especially with venlafaxine), serotonin syndrome, and the risk of **manic switch** in bipolar disorder patients, particularly when used without a mood stabilizer.
- **Drug Interactions:**
    - **With MAOIs:** Risk of serotonin syndrome.
    - **With NSAIDs and anticoagulants:** Increased risk of bleeding.
    - **With Lithium:** Can increase the risk of serotonin syndrome.

5.2.3. Mixed Episodes:

Mixed episodes feature simultaneous symptoms of mania and depression, making treatment particularly complex.

- **Valproate** is particularly effective in managing mixed episodes, as it helps reduce both manic and depressive symptoms.
- **Atypical antipsychotics** like **aripiprazole**, **quetiapine**, and **olanzapine** can also be used to stabilize mood during mixed episodes, helping reduce irritability and mood instability.

5.3. Maintenance Treatment Strategies

Once an acute episode has been stabilized, maintenance treatment aims to prevent relapse, reduce the frequency and severity of mood episodes, and improve overall functioning. Long-term maintenance often requires a combination of pharmacotherapy, psychotherapy, and lifestyle modifications.

1. Lithium:

- **Lithium** remains the gold standard for maintenance therapy in bipolar disorder, as it reduces the risk of both manic and depressive episodes and has a **suicide-preventive effect**. Regular monitoring of lithium levels is essential due to its narrow therapeutic index and risk of toxicity.

2. Valproate:

- **Valproate** is another commonly used maintenance medication, particularly effective for individuals with rapid cycling or mixed features.

3. Lamotrigine:

- **Lamotrigine** is particularly beneficial in preventing depressive episodes during maintenance treatment, though it is less effective for preventing mania .

4. Atypical Antipsychotics:

- **Quetiapine**, **aripiprazole**, and **olanzapine** are often used in maintenance therapy, especially for patients who have psychotic features or who have responded well to these medications during acute treatment .

5. Combination Therapy:

- Combination therapy may be necessary for individuals who do not respond adequately to monotherapy. For example, a mood stabilizer such as **lithium** may be combined with an atypical antipsychotic like **quetiapine** to provide more robust protection against mood swings.

6. Psychotherapy:

- **Cognitive Behavioral Therapy (CBT)** and **Psychoeducation** are important adjuncts to pharmacological treatment. Psychoeducation helps individuals and families recognize early signs of mood changes, adhere to medication, and implement lifestyle strategies to reduce the risk of relapse .
- **Interpersonal and Social Rhythm Therapy (IPSRT)** focuses on maintaining regular daily routines and sleep patterns, which can help stabilize mood in individuals with bipolar disorder .

7. Lifestyle Interventions:

- Encouraging **regular exercise**, a **balanced diet**, **good sleep hygiene**, and **stress management** can significantly reduce the likelihood of mood episodes. **Avoiding alcohol and substance use** is critical, as these can exacerbate symptoms and interfere with treatment.

Bipolar disorder is a complex condition that requires careful diagnosis and individualized treatment strategies for managing its different phases—mania, depression, and mixed episodes. Pharmacotherapy remains the cornerstone of treatment, with mood stabilizers, antipsychotics, and in some cases, antidepressants playing a key role in symptom management.

Maintenance treatment is essential to prevent relapse and promote long-term stability, and a comprehensive approach that includes pharmacological, psychological, and lifestyle interventions is most effective.

5.4. ICD-10 for Bipolar Disorder

The **ICD-10** codes for **Bipolar Disorder** are categorized based on the type and severity of the disorder.

- **F31.0**: Bipolar affective disorder, current episode hypomanic
- **F31.1**: Bipolar affective disorder, current episode manic without psychotic symptoms
- **F31.2**: Bipolar affective disorder, current episode manic with psychotic symptoms
- **F31.3**: Bipolar affective disorder, current episode mild or moderate depression
- **F31.4**: Bipolar affective disorder, current episode severe depression without psychotic symptoms
- **F31.5**: Bipolar affective disorder, current episode severe depression with psychotic symptoms
- **F31.6**: Bipolar affective disorder, current episode mixed
- **F31.7**: Bipolar affective disorder, currently in remission
- **F31.8**: Other bipolar affective disorders
- **F31.9**: Bipolar affective disorder, unspecified

References:

1. Geddes, J. R., & Miklowitz, D. J. (2013). Treatment of bipolar disorder. *The Lancet*, 381(9878), 1672-1682.
2. Malhi, G. S., Bellivier, F., Berk, M., et al. (2012). The bipolar spectrum. *Australian and New Zealand Journal of Psychiatry*, 46(2), 128-146.
3. Yatham, L. N., Kennedy, S. H., Parikh, S. V., et al. (2018). Canadian Network for Mood and Anxiety Treatments (CANMAT) and International Society for Bipolar Disorders (ISBD) 2018 guidelines for the management of patients with bipolar disorder. *Bipolar Disorders*, 20(2), 97-170.
4. Cipriani, A., Hawton, K., Stockton, S., & Geddes, J. R. (2013). Lithium in the prevention of suicide in mood disorders: Updated systematic review and meta-analysis. *BMJ*, 346, f3646.
5. Goodwin, G. M., Haddad, P. M., Ferrier, I. N., et al. (2016). Evidence-based guidelines for treating bipolar disorder: Revised third edition recommendations from the British Association for Psychopharmacology. *Journal of Psychopharmacology*, 30(6), 495-553.

Chapter 6: Anxiety Disorders

Anxiety disorders represent one of the most common categories of mental health conditions, characterized by excessive fear, worry, or nervousness that interferes with daily functioning. The major types of anxiety disorders include **Generalized Anxiety Disorder (GAD)**, **Panic Disorder**, **Social Anxiety Disorder (SAD)**, and **Specific Phobias**.

Treatment often involves a combination of pharmacotherapy and psychotherapy, with patient education playing a critical role in managing symptoms. This chapter covers the different types of anxiety disorders, explores **pharmacotherapy options**, and outlines **psychotherapy interventions** and **patient education** strategies.

6.1. Overview of Generalized Anxiety Disorder

6.1.1. Generalized Anxiety Disorder (GAD):

- GAD is characterized by **excessive, uncontrollable worry** about various aspects of life (e.g., work, health, relationships) that occurs on more days than not for at least six months. The worry is accompanied by at least three of the following symptoms: restlessness, fatigue, difficulty concentrating, irritability, muscle tension, and sleep disturbances .
- GAD is highly comorbid with other psychiatric conditions such as depression and often leads to significant impairment in daily functioning .

6.1.2. Panic Disorder:

- Panic disorder is defined by **recurrent, unexpected panic attacks**, which are sudden episodes of intense fear or discomfort accompanied by physical symptoms such as palpitations, sweating, chest pain, dizziness, and shortness of breath. Panic attacks are often followed by persistent concern about having another attack or changes in behavior to avoid potential triggers .
- Many individuals with panic disorder develop **agoraphobia**, a fear of situations in which escape might be difficult or help unavailable in the event of a panic attack, leading to avoidance of public places or travel .

6.1.3. Social Anxiety Disorder (SAD):

- SAD is characterized by a marked fear of **social or performance situations** in which the individual is exposed to potential scrutiny by others. The fear of embarrassment, humiliation, or rejection causes the person to avoid such situations or endure them with significant distress .
- SAD can severely limit an individual's ability to engage in work, education, and social activities, leading to isolation and reduced quality of life .

6.1.4. Specific Phobias:

- Specific phobias involve an intense, irrational fear of a specific object or situation (e.g., heights, animals, flying, needles) that leads to avoidance behaviors. The fear is out of proportion to the actual danger and causes significant distress or impairment .
- Exposure to the feared object or situation triggers an immediate anxiety response, which can manifest as a panic attack in some individuals .

6.2. Pharmacotherapy Options: Anxiolytics, Antidepressants, and Buspirone

Pharmacotherapy is an important component of anxiety disorder treatment, particularly for individuals with moderate to severe symptoms. The choice of medication depends on the type of anxiety disorder, the severity of symptoms, and the patient's comorbid conditions.

6.2.1. Anxiolytics (Benzodiazepines):

- **Benzodiazepines** (e.g., **alprazolam**, **lorazepam**, **diazepam**) are highly effective in reducing acute anxiety symptoms due to their rapid onset of action. They work by enhancing the activity of **gamma-aminobutyric acid (GABA)**, the brain's primary inhibitory neurotransmitter.
- While benzodiazepines are beneficial for short-term relief of acute anxiety or panic attacks, they are generally not recommended for long-term use due to the risks of **dependence**, **tolerance**, and **withdrawal**. Additionally, benzodiazepines can impair cognitive and psychomotor function, making them less suitable for individuals who require sustained daily treatment .
- **Clonazepam** and **lorazepam** are commonly used to treat panic disorder and GAD, but their use should be closely monitored .

6.2.2. Antidepressants:

- **Selective Serotonin Reuptake Inhibitors (SSRIs)**: SSRIs are considered first-line treatment for most anxiety disorders, including GAD, panic disorder, SAD, and specific phobias. Medications such as **sertraline**, **escitalopram**, and **paroxetine** increase serotonin levels in the brain, which can reduce anxiety symptoms over time . SSRIs are particularly effective for long-term management, although their therapeutic effects may take several weeks to become evident.
- **Serotonin-Norepinephrine Reuptake Inhibitors (SNRIs)**: SNRIs such as **venlafaxine** and **duloxetine** are also effective for treating anxiety disorders by increasing levels of both serotonin and norepinephrine. SNRIs are especially useful in individuals with comorbid depression and anxiety .
- **Tricyclic Antidepressants (TCAs)**: Although less commonly used due to their side effect profile, TCAs such as **clomipramine** can be effective in treating panic disorder and OCD. Their use is typically reserved for patients who have not responded to SSRIs or SNRIs .

6.2.3. Buspirone:

- **Buspirone** is an anxiolytic that acts as a partial agonist at serotonin **5-HT1A receptors**. Unlike benzodiazepines, buspirone does not cause sedation, dependence, or withdrawal, making it a safer option for long-term management of GAD. However, its onset of action is slower than that of benzodiazepines, and it is generally less effective in treating acute anxiety or panic attacks.

6.3. Psychotherapy and Cognitive-Behavioral Interventions

Psychotherapy, particularly **Cognitive-Behavioral Therapy (CBT)**, is a well-established, evidence-based treatment for anxiety disorders. CBT focuses on changing maladaptive thought patterns and behaviors that contribute to anxiety, helping patients develop coping strategies to manage their symptoms.

6.3.1. Cognitive-Behavioral Therapy (CBT):

- **CBT** is the gold standard of psychotherapy for anxiety disorders. It involves identifying and challenging irrational thoughts, or cognitive distortions, that contribute to anxiety (e.g., catastrophic thinking, overestimation of threat). CBT also includes **exposure therapy**, which gradually exposes patients to feared situations or objects in a controlled and systematic manner, reducing avoidance behaviors and desensitizing the individual to anxiety-provoking stimuli.
- CBT has been shown to be effective in treating a wide range of anxiety disorders, including GAD, panic disorder, SAD, and specific phobias. For example, exposure-based CBT is the most effective treatment for specific phobias, while cognitive restructuring techniques are particularly useful in SAD.

6.3.2. Acceptance and Commitment Therapy (ACT):

- **ACT** emphasizes accepting negative thoughts and feelings rather than trying to eliminate them. Patients learn to live with anxiety while engaging in valued life activities. ACT incorporates mindfulness techniques to reduce the distress caused by anxiety symptoms and enhance psychological flexibility.

6.3.3. Mindfulness-Based Stress Reduction (MBSR):

- **MBSR** is a structured program that teaches individuals mindfulness meditation techniques to manage anxiety. It has been shown to reduce anxiety symptoms by improving awareness of present-moment experiences and reducing rumination on fears about the future.

6.4. Patient Education and Counseling for Anxiety Management

Effective treatment of anxiety disorders requires comprehensive patient education and ongoing support. Counseling on lifestyle changes, medication adherence, and self-management strategies is crucial in helping patients achieve long-term anxiety control.

6.4.1. Medication Adherence and Expectations:

- Patients should be educated about the importance of **medication adherence**, especially with antidepressants, which may take several weeks to show their full therapeutic effect. They should also be informed about potential side effects and the risks of abrupt discontinuation, particularly with benzodiazepines .
- Patients taking SSRIs or SNRIs may experience transient side effects such as nausea, headache, or sexual dysfunction, which typically resolve over time. Encouraging adherence despite early side effects can improve long-term outcomes.

6.4.2. Stress Management Techniques:

- Teaching patients **stress management** techniques such as **deep breathing**, **progressive muscle relaxation**, and **guided imagery** can provide immediate relief from acute anxiety symptoms. These techniques are particularly useful during high-stress situations, such as social events or public speaking for individuals with SAD .
- **Exercise** has also been shown to reduce anxiety symptoms by releasing endorphins and improving mood. Encouraging patients to incorporate regular physical activity into their routine can complement pharmacotherapy and psychotherapy .

6.4.3. Sleep Hygiene:

- Anxiety disorders are often associated with **sleep disturbances**, including insomnia. Educating patients on **good sleep hygiene** practices, such as maintaining a regular sleep schedule, limiting caffeine intake, and creating a relaxing bedtime routine, can help reduce anxiety and improve overall well-being .

6.4.4. Avoidance of Stimulants:

- Patients with anxiety disorders should be advised to **limit or avoid stimulants** such as **caffeine**, **nicotine**, and **illicit drugs**, as these substances can exacerbate anxiety symptoms and interfere with sleep .

6.4.5. Support Systems for General Anxiety Disorders:

- Encouraging patients to seek **social support** from family, friends, or support groups can reduce isolation and provide emotional support. Involvement in group therapy can also provide a sense of community and shared understanding, particularly for individuals with social anxiety disorder .

Anxiety disorders are highly prevalent and can significantly impair an individual's quality of life. Treatment often involves a combination of pharmacotherapy (including SSRIs, SNRIs, and benzodiazepines) and psychotherapy, particularly CBT.

Educating patients on medication adherence, stress management, and lifestyle modifications plays a crucial role in the successful management of anxiety. Long-term outcomes are improved when patients are actively involved in their treatment and equipped with tools to manage their symptoms effectively.

6.5. ICD-10 for Anxiety Disorders

These codes cover a wide range of **anxiety-related disorders**, helping healthcare providers classify and diagnose various forms of anxiety for appropriate treatment and management.

1. **F41.1 – Generalized Anxiety Disorder (GAD)**
   - Characterized by excessive worry and anxiety about various aspects of life, such as work, social interactions, and everyday situations, which lasts for six months or more.
2. **F41.0 – Panic Disorder (episodic paroxysmal anxiety)**
   - Recurrent unexpected panic attacks that cause ongoing concern or behavioral changes due to fear of future attacks.
3. **F40.00 – Agoraphobia without Panic Disorder**
   - Fear or anxiety about situations where escape might be difficult, such as being in open spaces, crowds, or public transportation, without a history of panic disorder.
4. **F40.10 – Social Phobia (Social Anxiety Disorder)**
   - A significant and persistent fear of social or performance situations where there is exposure to possible scrutiny by others, leading to avoidance behaviors.
5. **F40.218 – Specific Phobia, Other**
   - Intense fear or anxiety triggered by a specific object or situation (e.g., flying, heights, animals), leading to avoidance or significant distress.
6. **F43.10 – Post-Traumatic Stress Disorder (PTSD), Unspecified**
   - Anxiety symptoms that occur after exposure to a traumatic event, such as flashbacks, avoidance of trauma-related stimuli, hypervigilance, and intrusive memories.
7. **F43.0 – Acute Stress Reaction**
   - Transient anxiety and emotional disturbance that develops in response to an exceptional physical or psychological stressor and resolves within a few days.
8. **F41.8 – Other Specified Anxiety Disorders**
   - Anxiety disorders that don't fully meet the criteria for a specific disorder but are still clinically significant (e.g., mixed anxiety-depressive disorder).
9. **F41.9 – Anxiety Disorder, Unspecified**
   - Used when the specific anxiety disorder cannot be determined or doesn't fit neatly into any other anxiety category.
10. **F40.230 – Claustrophobia**
- A specific phobia characterized by a fear of being in enclosed or confined spaces.

References:

1. American Psychiatric Association. (2013). *Diagnostic and Statistical Manual of Mental Disorders* (5th ed.).
2. Baldwin, D. S., Anderson, I. M., Nutt, D. J., et al. (2014). Evidence-based pharmacological treatment of anxiety disorders, post-traumatic stress disorder and obsessive-compulsive disorder: A revision of the 2005 guidelines from the British Association for Psychopharmacology. *Journal of Psychopharmacology*, 28(5), 403-439.
3. Bandelow, B., Reitt, M., Röver, C., et al. (2015). Efficacy of treatments for anxiety disorders: A meta-analysis. *International Clinical Psychopharmacology*, 30(4), 183-192.
4. Hofmann, S. G., Asnaani, A., Vonk, I. J., et al. (2012). The efficacy of cognitive behavioral therapy: A review of meta-analyses. *Cognitive Therapy and Research*, 36(5), 427-440.
5. Wetherell, J. L., Gatz, M., & Craske, M. G. (2003). Treatment of generalized anxiety disorder in older adults. *Journal of Anxiety Disorders*, 17(3), 299-317.
6. Otto, M. W., & Pollack, M. H. (2009). The role of psychotherapy in the treatment of anxiety disorders. *Journal of Clinical Psychiatry*, 70(Suppl 2), 10-16.

Chapter 7: Schizophrenia and Other Psychotic Disorders

Schizophrenia and related psychotic disorders are severe mental health conditions that significantly impair a person's ability to think clearly, manage emotions, make decisions, and relate to others. Understanding these disorders, as well as the pharmacological and non-pharmacological treatments, is critical for effective management.

This chapter explores the **psychotic spectrum**, reviews **antipsychotic medications** (first- and second-generation), discusses their **adverse effects and monitoring considerations**, and examines both **pharmacological and non-pharmacological approaches** to managing psychosis.

7.1. Understanding the Psychotic Spectrum

Psychotic disorders are characterized by abnormalities in thinking and perception, often leading to **hallucinations**, **delusions**, **disorganized thinking**, and impaired reality testing. Schizophrenia is the most prominent disorder on the psychotic spectrum, but other conditions are also categorized under this group.

7.1.1. Schizophrenia:

- Schizophrenia is a chronic disorder characterized by **positive symptoms** (e.g., hallucinations, delusions, disorganized speech), **negative symptoms** (e.g., flat affect, social withdrawal, lack of motivation), and **cognitive deficits** (e.g., impaired attention, memory, and executive function) . To meet the DSM-5 criteria for schizophrenia, a patient must experience at least **two or more symptoms** for at least **six months**, with at least one of the symptoms being delusions, hallucinations, or disorganized speech .
- Schizophrenia affects approximately 1% of the global population and typically presents in late adolescence or early adulthood. The course of the disorder is often chronic, with episodic exacerbations of psychotic symptoms .

7.1.2. Schizoaffective Disorder:

- Schizoaffective disorder combines features of schizophrenia and mood disorders. Patients experience symptoms of schizophrenia along with prominent mood episodes (depression or mania). To be diagnosed, patients must have a period of illness during which they experience psychotic symptoms for at least **two weeks** without mood symptoms, followed by periods with both psychosis and mood disturbance .

7.1.3. Brief Psychotic Disorder:

- This disorder is characterized by the sudden onset of psychotic symptoms (e.g., hallucinations, delusions) lasting at least one day but less than one month, followed by full remission and return to normal functioning. Brief psychotic disorder is often precipitated by extreme stress or trauma .

7.1.4. Delusional Disorder:

- Delusional disorder involves the presence of **non-bizarre delusions** (i.e., beliefs that could plausibly occur in real life) for at least one month without the presence of other psychotic symptoms, such as hallucinations or disorganized thinking .

7.1.5. Substance-Induced Psychotic Disorder:

- Psychotic symptoms can be triggered by intoxication or withdrawal from substances such as alcohol, cannabis, stimulants, or hallucinogens. The symptoms typically resolve once the substance use is discontinued .

7.2. Antipsychotic Medications: First-Generation vs. Second-Generation Agents

Antipsychotic medications are the cornerstone of treatment for schizophrenia and other psychotic disorders. They are divided into two categories: **first-generation antipsychotics (FGAs)** and **second-generation antipsychotics (SGAs)**, also known as **typical** and **atypical antipsychotics**, respectively. These medications target the **dopamine D2 receptors**, with newer agents also affecting **serotonin receptors**.

7.2.1. First-Generation Antipsychotics (FGAs):

- **FGAs**, such as **haloperidol**, **chlorpromazine**, and **fluphenazine**, primarily block **dopamine D2 receptors**, leading to a reduction in positive symptoms (hallucinations, delusions) but with a higher risk of **extrapyramidal side effects (EPS)**.
- **Haloperidol** is one of the most commonly used FGAs and is highly effective in controlling acute psychotic symptoms. However, FGAs are associated with significant side effects, including **tardive dyskinesia** (involuntary movements), **parkinsonism**, and **akathisia** (restlessness), which limit their use, especially in the long term .

7.2.2. Second-Generation Antipsychotics (SGAs):

- **SGAs**, such as **risperidone, olanzapine, quetiapine**, and **aripiprazole**, block both **dopamine D2 receptors** and **serotonin 5-HT2A receptors**, which helps reduce both **positive** and **negative** symptoms with a lower risk of EPS compared to FGAs.
- SGAs have become the first-line treatment for schizophrenia due to their more favorable side effect profile. For example, **aripiprazole** is known for its relatively low metabolic side effects, while **olanzapine** and **clozapine** are more effective in treatment-resistant schizophrenia but are associated with significant metabolic risks, such as **weight gain**, **hyperlipidemia**, and **diabetes** .

- **Clozapine** is particularly effective in patients with **treatment-resistant schizophrenia** and those at risk of **suicide**, but its use is limited by the risk of **agranulocytosis** (a potentially life-threatening drop in white blood cells), necessitating regular blood monitoring.

7.3. Adverse Effects of Medications and Monitoring Considerations

Both FGAs and SGAs carry a range of potential adverse effects, and careful monitoring is essential to ensure the safety and well-being of patients.

7.3.1. Extrapyramidal Side Effects (EPS):

- FGAs are more likely to cause **extrapyramidal side effects**, which include **dystonia** (muscle spasms), **akathisia**, **parkinsonism**, and **tardive dyskinesia**. These side effects are caused by excessive dopamine blockade in the **nigrostriatal pathway**.
- Treatment for EPS may include lowering the dose of the antipsychotic or adding medications such as **benztropine** (an anticholinergic) or **beta-blockers** to reduce symptoms.

7.3.2. Metabolic Side Effects:

- SGAs are associated with **metabolic syndrome**, which includes **weight gain**, **hyperglycemia**, **insulin resistance**, and **dyslipidemia**. Patients taking SGAs, especially **clozapine** and **olanzapine**, should have their **weight**, **lipid profile**, and **blood glucose levels** monitored regularly.
- Lifestyle interventions, such as diet and exercise, are recommended to mitigate these risks. In some cases, switching to an SGA with a lower metabolic risk profile (e.g., **aripiprazole** or **lurasidone**) may be necessary.

7.3.3. Cardiovascular Risks:

- Both FGAs and SGAs can prolong the **QT interval**, increasing the risk of potentially life-threatening arrhythmias like **torsades de pointes**. Regular **electrocardiogram (ECG)** monitoring is recommended, especially in patients taking FGAs or SGAs known to have higher cardiac risk (e.g., **haloperidol** or **ziprasidone**).

7.3.4. Agranulocytosis:

- **Clozapine** requires special monitoring due to the risk of **agranulocytosis**, a serious condition that reduces the number of white blood cells, increasing the risk of infection. Patients on clozapine must have regular **complete blood count (CBC)** monitoring according to a strict protocol (e.g., weekly for the first six months, then every two weeks).

7.4. Pharmacological and Non-Pharmacological Approaches to Managing Psychosis

7.4.1. Pharmacological Approaches:

- **Antipsychotic Maintenance Therapy**: Most patients with schizophrenia require long-term antipsychotic treatment to prevent relapse. SGAs are generally preferred for maintenance therapy due to their better tolerability. **Long-acting injectable (LAI) antipsychotics** (e.g., **paliperidone palmitate**, **aripiprazole LAI**) are often used to improve adherence in patients who struggle with daily oral medication .
- **Adjunctive Medications**: In some cases, adjunctive medications may be added to antipsychotic therapy to address specific symptoms or side effects. For example, **benzodiazepines** can help manage agitation or anxiety, and **mood stabilizers** (e.g., **lithium**, **valproate**) may be used in patients with **schizoaffective disorder** or those who exhibit mood instability .

7.4.2. Non-Pharmacological Approaches:

- **Cognitive Behavioral Therapy for Psychosis (CBTp)**: **CBTp** is an evidence-based therapy that helps patients challenge distorted thoughts and beliefs related to psychotic experiences (e.g., hallucinations and delusions). It has been shown to reduce symptom severity and improve functioning when used alongside antipsychotic medication .
- **Family Intervention**: Psychoeducation for families is essential to help them understand the nature of schizophrenia, improve communication, and reduce **expressed emotion** (e.g., criticism, hostility), which can reduce the risk of relapse .
- **Social Skills Training**: Schizophrenia often leads to impaired social functioning, and social skills training can help individuals improve interpersonal communication, vocational functioning, and daily living skills .
- **Assertive Community Treatment (ACT)**: **ACT** is an intensive, team-based approach that provides comprehensive, individualized support to individuals with severe schizophrenia. The goal is to keep patients stable and engaged in the community, reducing hospitalizations and improving quality of life .

Schizophrenia and other psychotic disorders present significant challenges, but with appropriate management, patients can achieve stability and improved functioning. Antipsychotic medications, particularly second-generation agents, are the cornerstone of treatment, but they must be used cautiously due to potential side effects. Non-pharmacological interventions, such as CBT for psychosis and family support, are essential adjuncts to pharmacotherapy. By addressing both the biological and psychosocial aspects of psychosis, comprehensive treatment plans can reduce the burden of these conditions on patients and their families.

7.5. ICD-10 for Schizophrenia and Related Psychotic Disorders

These codes cover various subtypes of schizophrenia and related psychotic disorders. Each diagnosis corresponds to specific clinical features or presentations within the psychotic spectrum.

Schizophrenia (F20 series):

- **F20.0** – Paranoid schizophrenia
- **F20.1** – Disorganized schizophrenia (hebephrenic)
- **F20.2** – Catatonic schizophrenia
- **F20.3** – Undifferentiated schizophrenia
- **F20.5** – Residual schizophrenia
- **F20.81** – Schizophreniform disorder
- **F20.89** – Other schizophrenia
- **F20.9** – Schizophrenia, unspecified

Other Psychotic Disorders:

- **F22** – Delusional disorders
- **F23** – Brief psychotic disorder
- **F24** – Shared psychotic disorder (Folie à deux)
- **F25.0** – Schizoaffective disorder, bipolar type
- **F25.1** – Schizoaffective disorder, depressive type
- **F25.8** – Other schizoaffective disorders
- **F25.9** – Schizoaffective disorder, unspecified
- **F28** – Other psychotic disorder not due to a substance or known physiological condition
- **F29** – Unspecified psychosis not due to a substance or known physiological condition

References:

1. American Psychiatric Association. (2013). *Diagnostic and Statistical Manual of Mental Disorders* (5th ed.).
2. Howes, O. D., & Kapur, S. (2009). The dopamine hypothesis of schizophrenia: Version III—The final common pathway. *Schizophrenia Bulletin*, 35(3), 549-562.
3. Lieberman, J. A., Stroup, T. S., McEvoy, J. P., et al. (2005). Effectiveness of antipsychotic drugs in patients with chronic schizophrenia. *New England Journal of Medicine*, 353(12), 1209-1223.
4. Leucht, S., Cipriani, A., Spineli, L., et al. (2013). Comparative efficacy and tolerability of 15 antipsychotic drugs in schizophrenia: A multiple-treatments meta-analysis. *The Lancet*, 382(9896), 951-962.
5. Kane, J. M., Correll, C. U., & Citrome, L. (2013). Guidelines for the management of schizophrenia: A focus on long-acting injectable antipsychotics. *CNS Drugs*, 27(9), 749-762.
6. Morrison, A. P., Turkington, D., Pyle, M., et al. (2014). Cognitive therapy for people with schizophrenia spectrum disorders not taking antipsychotic drugs: A single-blind randomized controlled trial. *The Lancet*, 383(9926), 1395-1403.

Chapter 8: Attention-Deficit/Hyperactivity Disorder (ADHD)

Attention-Deficit/Hyperactivity Disorder (ADHD) is a neurodevelopmental disorder characterized by persistent patterns of **inattention**, **hyperactivity**, and **impulsivity** that impair daily functioning. ADHD is one of the most common childhood psychiatric disorders and can persist into adolescence and adulthood.

This chapter covers the **overview of ADHD**, **diagnostic criteria**, **pharmacotherapy options**, the importance of **patient education** on medication adherence and lifestyle modifications, and the role of **collaborative care** in managing ADHD.

8.1. Overview of ADHD and Diagnostic Criteria

ADHD is primarily diagnosed during childhood, with symptoms typically appearing before the age of 12. However, it can continue into adolescence and adulthood, affecting daily activities such as academic performance, work, and relationships. According to the **DSM-5**, ADHD is categorized into three types:

1. **Predominantly Inattentive Presentation** (previously known as ADD):
   - Individuals exhibit symptoms of inattention (e.g., difficulty maintaining focus, disorganization) without significant hyperactivity or impulsivity.
2. **Predominantly Hyperactive-Impulsive Presentation**:
   - Individuals demonstrate excessive energy, hyperactivity (e.g., fidgeting, inability to stay seated), and impulsive behavior (e.g., difficulty waiting their turn).
3. **Combined Presentation**:
   - Individuals show a mix of inattentive and hyperactive-impulsive symptoms.

8.2. DSM-5 Diagnostic Criteria for ADHD:

To meet the diagnostic criteria, children must display at least **six symptoms** (or five for adolescents/adults over 17 years) from the following categories, for at least **six months**:

- **Inattention**:
  - Fails to give close attention to details or makes careless mistakes.
  - Difficulty sustaining attention in tasks or play.
  - Does not seem to listen when spoken to directly.
  - Does not follow through on instructions and fails to finish tasks.
  - Difficulty organizing tasks and activities.
  - Avoids tasks that require sustained mental effort.
  - Often loses things necessary for tasks or activities.
  - Easily distracted by extraneous stimuli.
  - Often forgetful in daily activities.
- **Hyperactivity-Impulsivity**:

- Fidgets with hands or feet or squirms in seat.
- Leaves seat when remaining seated is expected.
- Runs or climbs in inappropriate situations (in adults, may feel restless).
- Unable to play quietly.
- "On the go" or acts as if "driven by a motor."
- Talks excessively.
- Blurts out answers before questions have been completed.
- Difficulty waiting for their turn.
- Interrupts or intrudes on others.

These symptoms must cause significant impairment in **social**, **academic**, or **occupational functioning** and cannot be better explained by another mental health condition, such as an anxiety disorder or mood disorder.

8.3. Pharmacotherapy Options: Stimulants, Non-Stimulants, and Alpha-2 Agonists

Pharmacotherapy is the most widely used and effective treatment for managing ADHD, especially when combined with behavioral interventions. Medications for ADHD fall into three main categories: **stimulants**, **non-stimulants**, and **alpha-2 agonists**.

8.3.1. Stimulants:

Stimulants are the first-line treatment for ADHD and are highly effective in reducing both inattentive and hyperactive-impulsive symptoms. Stimulants work by increasing levels of **dopamine** and **norepinephrine** in the brain, which improves attention, focus, and impulse control.

- **Methylphenidate**: This is one of the most commonly prescribed stimulants for ADHD and includes both immediate-release (IR) and extended-release (ER) formulations (e.g., **Ritalin**, **Concerta**, **Metadate**). Methylphenidate is effective for both children and adults with ADHD, with effects noticeable within 30-60 minutes of administration .
- **Amphetamines**: Amphetamine-based stimulants, including **dextroamphetamine** (e.g., **Dexedrine**) and **mixed amphetamine salts** (e.g., **Adderall**, **Vyvanse**), are also widely used for ADHD. Like methylphenidate, amphetamines increase dopamine and norepinephrine availability in the brain, enhancing focus and reducing hyperactivity .

Side Effects of Stimulants: Common side effects include **decreased appetite**, **insomnia**, **headache**, **irritability**, and **increased heart rate** or **blood pressure**. In rare cases, stimulants may exacerbate tics or anxiety. Growth retardation can occur with long-term use in children, so periodic assessment of growth and weight is recommended .

8.3.2. Non-Stimulants:

Non-stimulant medications are typically used when stimulants are ineffective or not tolerated due to side effects. These medications have a different mechanism of action and tend to have a slower onset.

- **Atomoxetine (Strattera)**: Atomoxetine is a selective **norepinephrine reuptake inhibitor** (NRI) and is FDA-approved for the treatment of ADHD. It is effective in reducing inattention and hyperactivity, though its effects may take several weeks to manifest. Atomoxetine is less likely to cause insomnia or appetite suppression compared to stimulants .
- **Bupropion**: Though primarily an antidepressant, **bupropion** is sometimes used off-label for ADHD, particularly in patients who have comorbid depression. It acts as a **dopamine-norepinephrine reuptake inhibitor (DNRI)** and can improve attention and impulse control .

8.3.3. Alpha-2 Agonists:

Alpha-2 adrenergic agonists are often used as adjuncts to stimulants or as alternative treatments for ADHD, particularly in children who experience excessive hyperactivity, impulsivity, or aggression.

- **Clonidine**: This medication reduces hyperactivity and impulsivity by stimulating **alpha-2 adrenergic receptors** in the brain, leading to a calming effect. It is often used in combination with stimulants to reduce impulsivity and aggression .
- **Guanfacine**: Another alpha-2 agonist, guanfacine (e.g., **Intuniv**) is approved for the treatment of ADHD and is particularly effective in managing hyperactive and impulsive symptoms. It is also less sedating than clonidine and has a longer duration of action .

8.4. Patient Education on Medication Adherence and Lifestyle Modifications

Effective management of ADHD requires patient and caregiver education on medication adherence, the importance of lifestyle changes, and the need for ongoing behavioral support.

8.4.1. Medication Adherence:

- **Education on Dosing and Timing**: Patients should be informed about the importance of taking medications at the prescribed times, especially for stimulant medications, where improper timing can affect sleep or appetite. Extended-release formulations may be preferable for individuals who need all-day symptom control, while immediate-release formulations may require multiple daily doses .
- **Monitoring for Side Effects**: Patients and caregivers should be educated on the potential side effects of ADHD medications (e.g., decreased appetite, insomnia) and the importance of communicating these issues to the prescribing physician. Regular monitoring of weight, height (in children), and vital signs (heart rate and blood pressure) is important to detect any adverse effects early .
- **Managing Missed Doses**: Clear guidance should be provided on what to do if a dose is missed, particularly with stimulants. Missing doses can lead to fluctuations in symptoms, which can affect daily functioning .

8.4.2. Lifestyle Modifications:

- **Sleep Hygiene**: Many individuals with ADHD, especially those taking stimulants, struggle with sleep difficulties. Educating patients about good sleep hygiene (e.g., maintaining a consistent sleep schedule, reducing caffeine intake, creating a relaxing bedtime routine) is essential for managing both ADHD symptoms and medication side effects .
- **Diet and Exercise**: Regular physical activity can help reduce hyperactivity and improve focus. A balanced diet rich in nutrients is also important for overall health and well-being. Stimulants can suppress appetite, so ensuring proper nutrition is key, particularly for children .
- **Structured Routines**: Establishing daily routines, such as consistent schedules for homework, chores, and leisure activities, can help reduce disorganization and improve time management. Behavioral strategies such as reward systems for task completion can also enhance adherence to routines .

8.5. Collaborative Care with Other Healthcare Providers in Managing ADHD

Managing ADHD effectively requires a **multidisciplinary approach**, with collaboration between physicians, psychologists, educators, and other healthcare providers.

8.5.1. Role of Psychologists and Behavioral Therapists:

- **Behavioral Interventions**: Cognitive-behavioral therapy (CBT) and behavioral interventions are effective non-pharmacological treatments for ADHD. These therapies help individuals with ADHD develop skills to manage impulsivity, improve organization, and enhance emotional regulation .
- **Parent and Teacher Training**: Educating parents and teachers about ADHD and effective behavioral management strategies is critical for improving a child's functioning at home and school. Behavioral interventions such as positive reinforcement and clear, consistent rules can significantly improve outcomes for children with ADHD .

8.5.2. Coordination with Schools and Educators:

- **Individualized Education Plans (IEPs)**: Many children with ADHD benefit from IEPs, which are tailored to their unique learning needs. Teachers and school staff play a key role in implementing accommodations, such as extra time on tests, seating arrangements, and breaks during lessons .
- **Communication between Healthcare Providers and Schools**: Regular communication between healthcare providers, parents, and schools ensures that the child's academic and behavioral needs are addressed consistently. Teachers can provide valuable feedback on the child's behavior and performance in the classroom, which can help inform treatment decisions .

8.5.3. Involvement of Pediatricians and Primary Care Providers:

- **Routine Monitoring**: Pediatricians and primary care providers are essential for routine monitoring of growth, vital signs, and potential side effects of medications. They also serve as the first point of contact for addressing concerns related to ADHD treatment .
- **Management of Comorbid Conditions**: Many individuals with ADHD also have comorbid conditions such as anxiety, depression, or learning disabilities. Collaborative care ensures that these conditions are properly managed alongside ADHD, improving overall functioning .

ADHD is a complex neurodevelopmental disorder that requires a comprehensive treatment approach. Pharmacotherapy, particularly stimulants, plays a key role in managing symptoms, but non-stimulant medications and alpha-2 agonists provide alternatives when stimulants are not suitable. Patient education on medication adherence and lifestyle modifications is crucial to treatment success, and collaborative care with psychologists, educators, and primary care providers is essential for addressing the broader needs of individuals with ADHD. Through a combination of pharmacological and behavioral interventions, most individuals with ADHD can achieve significant improvements in functioning and quality of life.

8.6. ICD-10 for ADHD

These codes differentiate between the various presentations of ADHD based on the predominant symptoms (inattentive, hyperactive-impulsive, or combined), as well as other or unspecified types.

- **F90.0** – Attention-deficit hyperactivity disorder, predominantly inattentive type
- **F90.1** – Attention-deficit hyperactivity disorder, predominantly hyperactive-impulsive type
- **F90.2** – Attention-deficit hyperactivity disorder, combined type
- **F90.8** – Other attention-deficit hyperactivity disorders
- **F90.9** – Attention-deficit hyperactivity disorder, unspecified

References:

1. American Psychiatric Association. (2013). *Diagnostic and Statistical Manual of Mental Disorders* (5th ed.).
2. Faraone, S. V., Biederman, J., & Mick, E. (2006). The age-dependent decline of attention deficit hyperactivity disorder: A meta-analysis of follow-up studies. *Psychological Medicine*, 36(2), 159-165.
3. Cortese, S. (2020). Pharmacologic treatment of attention deficit-hyperactivity disorder. *New England Journal of Medicine*, 383(11), 1050-1056.
4. Banaschewski, T., Gerlach, M., Becker, K., et al. (2013). Non-stimulant medications in the treatment of ADHD. *European Child & Adolescent Psychiatry*, 22(1), S15-S23.
5. Hinshaw, S. P., & Arnold, L. E. (2015). Attention-deficit hyperactivity disorder, multimodal treatment, and longitudinal outcome: Evidence, paradox, and challenge. *Wiley Interdisciplinary Reviews: Cognitive Science*, 6(1), 39-52.
6. Pliszka, S. R., & the AACAP Work Group on Quality Issues. (2007). Practice parameter for the assessment and treatment of children and adolescents with attention-deficit/hyperactivity disorder. *Journal of the American Academy of Child & Adolescent Psychiatry*, 46(7), 894-921.

Chapter 9: Substance Use Disorders

Substance use disorders (SUDs) are chronic, relapsing conditions characterized by compulsive substance seeking and use despite harmful consequences. SUDs can lead to significant physical, psychological, and social impairments, making effective treatment essential.

This chapter provides an **overview of substance use disorders and addiction**, explores **pharmacotherapy options** for specific substances (alcohol, opioids, nicotine, and stimulants), examines **harm reduction strategies** and **medication-assisted treatment (MAT)**, and discusses the importance of **addressing stigma and promoting recovery**.

9.1. Overview of Substance Use Disorders and Addiction

9.1.1. Definition and Diagnostic Criteria:

According to the **DSM-5**, SUDs are defined by a maladaptive pattern of substance use leading to clinically significant impairment or distress, as manifested by **at least two** of the following criteria within a **12-month period**:

- Larger amounts of the substance are consumed than intended.
- Persistent desire or unsuccessful efforts to cut down or control use.
- Significant time is spent in activities to obtain, use, or recover from the substance.
- Craving or a strong desire to use the substance.
- Recurrent use results in failure to fulfill major obligations at work, school, or home.
- Continued use despite persistent social or interpersonal problems caused by the substance.
- Important social, occupational, or recreational activities are reduced or given up.
- Recurrent use in physically hazardous situations (e.g., driving under the influence).
- Continued use despite knowledge of a physical or psychological problem caused by the substance.
- **Tolerance** (increased amounts needed to achieve the desired effect).
- **Withdrawal** (development of a substance-specific syndrome upon cessation of use) .

9.1.2. The Neurobiology of Addiction:

Addiction is a brain disorder that involves alterations in the **reward, motivation, memory**, and **control** circuits of the brain. **Dopamine**, a neurotransmitter associated with pleasure and reward, plays a key role in the development of addiction. Substance use increases dopamine levels in the **mesolimbic pathway**, reinforcing the behavior and leading to repeated use despite negative consequences . Over time, the brain's reward system becomes less responsive to natural rewards, and individuals require increasing amounts of the substance to achieve the same effect (**tolerance**).

9.1.3. The Continuum of Substance Use:

Substance use exists on a continuum, ranging from **occasional or social use** to **problematic use** and ultimately **addiction**. Not everyone who uses substances develops a disorder, but the risk of SUD increases with **genetic**, **environmental**, and **psychosocial factors**, including exposure to trauma, stress, and early initiation of substance use.

9.2 Pharmacotherapy Options for Alcohol, Opioid, Nicotine, and Stimulant Use Disorders

Pharmacotherapy is a key component of treatment for many types of SUDs. Medications can help reduce cravings, manage withdrawal symptoms, and prevent relapse.

9.2.1. Alcohol Use Disorder:

- **Disulfiram (Antabuse)**: Disulfiram works by inhibiting the enzyme **aldehyde dehydrogenase**, leading to an accumulation of acetaldehyde when alcohol is consumed, causing unpleasant symptoms (e.g., flushing, nausea, vomiting). This creates a deterrent to drinking.
- **Naltrexone (Revia, Vivitrol)**: Naltrexone is an **opioid receptor antagonist** that reduces the pleasurable effects of alcohol and decreases cravings. It can be administered orally or as a monthly intramuscular injection (Vivitrol).
- **Acamprosate (Campral)**: Acamprosate helps reduce alcohol cravings by restoring the balance between **glutamate** and **GABA** neurotransmitter systems, which are dysregulated in individuals with alcohol dependence.

9.2.2. Opioid Use Disorder:

- **Methadone**: Methadone is a long-acting **opioid agonist** used in medication-assisted treatment (MAT) for opioid dependence. It reduces withdrawal symptoms and cravings without causing the euphoric effects of short-acting opioids like heroin.
- **Buprenorphine (Suboxone)**: Buprenorphine is a **partial opioid agonist** that binds to opioid receptors but with less intense effects compared to full agonists like methadone. It is often combined with **naloxone** (as in Suboxone) to prevent misuse.
- **Naltrexone**: In opioid use disorder, naltrexone blocks the effects of opioids, preventing euphoria if the patient relapses. It is particularly useful for individuals who have already detoxified from opioids and are motivated to remain abstinent.
- **Naloxone (Narcan)**: Naloxone is an **opioid antagonist** used to reverse opioid overdoses. It can rapidly restore normal respiration in individuals experiencing opioid overdose and is available as a nasal spray or injection.

9.2.3. Nicotine Use Disorder:

- **Nicotine Replacement Therapy (NRT)**: NRT products, including **nicotine patches**, **gum**, **lozenges**, **inhalers**, and **nasal sprays**, help reduce withdrawal symptoms and cravings by providing a controlled amount of nicotine without the harmful chemicals found in tobacco smoke .
- **Varenicline (Chantix)**: Varenicline is a **partial agonist at nicotine receptors** that reduces cravings and the pleasurable effects of smoking. It is highly effective in promoting smoking cessation .
- **Bupropion (Zyban)**: Originally developed as an antidepressant, bupropion is also used to reduce nicotine cravings and withdrawal symptoms. It works by inhibiting the reuptake of **dopamine** and **norepinephrine**, which are involved in nicotine addiction .

9.2.4. Stimulant Use Disorder (Cocaine, Amphetamines):

- There are currently no FDA-approved pharmacotherapies specifically for stimulant use disorder, though several medications are being investigated. However, certain **off-label medications** may be used to reduce cravings and manage withdrawal symptoms.
    - **Modafinil**: Modafinil, a wakefulness-promoting agent, has shown some promise in reducing cocaine use by affecting dopamine and glutamate systems.
    - **Topiramate**: This anticonvulsant has been studied for its potential to reduce cocaine cravings by modulating **GABA** and **glutamate** neurotransmission .
    - **Antidepressants**: In some cases, **SSRIs** or **bupropion** are used to manage mood symptoms or reduce cravings associated with stimulant use.

9.3. Harm Reduction Strategies and Medication-Assisted Treatment

9.3.1. Harm Reduction Strategies:

Harm reduction approaches aim to minimize the negative consequences of substance use without necessarily requiring complete abstinence. These strategies acknowledge that some individuals may continue to use substances but can do so in a way that reduces harm.

- **Needle Exchange Programs**: These programs provide clean syringes to individuals who inject drugs, reducing the transmission of **HIV**, **hepatitis C**, and other bloodborne infections .
- **Supervised Injection Sites**: These sites allow individuals to inject drugs in a medically supervised environment, reducing the risk of overdose and providing access to health services .
- **Naloxone Distribution**: Widespread distribution of **naloxone** kits to people at risk of opioid overdose, their friends, family members, and first responders has been shown to reduce overdose deaths .

9.3.2. Medication-Assisted Treatment (MAT):

MAT combines the use of medications (e.g., methadone, buprenorphine, naltrexone) with counseling and behavioral therapies to treat SUDs. It is particularly effective in treating **opioid use disorder** but can also be used in alcohol and nicotine use disorders.

- MAT has been shown to reduce **opioid use**, decrease the risk of **overdose**, improve **retention in treatment**, and reduce **criminal activity** among individuals with opioid use disorder .
- A common misconception is that MAT replaces one addiction with another, but research demonstrates that MAT significantly improves outcomes for individuals with opioid addiction by stabilizing brain chemistry and reducing the harmful behaviors associated with opioid misuse .

9.4. Addressing Stigma and Promoting Recovery in Substance Use Disorder Management

9.4.1. Addressing Stigma:

Stigma remains a significant barrier to effective treatment for individuals with SUDs. It can lead to social isolation, discrimination, and reluctance to seek help. **Healthcare providers**, **families**, and **society** play important roles in reducing stigma and supporting individuals in their recovery journey.

- **Person-First Language**: Encouraging the use of person-first language (e.g., "person with substance use disorder" rather than "addict" or "alcoholic") helps shift the focus from the individual's identity being defined by their disorder .
- **Education**: Educating the public and healthcare providers about the neurobiological basis of addiction can help reduce stigma and promote a more compassionate approach to treatment.

9.4.2. Promoting Recovery:

Recovery from SUD is a lifelong process that involves more than just abstinence from substances; it encompasses improvements in physical, psychological, and social well-being.

- **Peer Support**: Peer support groups, such as **Alcoholics Anonymous (AA)**, **Narcotics Anonymous (NA)**, and **SMART Recovery**, provide individuals with a supportive community of individuals in recovery, which has been shown to improve long-term outcomes .
- **Comprehensive Care**: Effective recovery programs incorporate not only pharmacotherapy and behavioral interventions but also services such as **housing support**, **vocational training**, and **mental health care** to address the social determinants of health that contribute to substance use.

Substance use disorders are complex, chronic conditions that require a multifaceted treatment approach. Pharmacotherapy plays a central role in managing cravings and preventing relapse for alcohol, opioid, and nicotine use disorders, while harm reduction strategies help reduce the negative consequences of substance use. Medication-assisted treatment has proven to be effective in treating opioid use disorder, but addressing the stigma associated with SUDs is equally important in promoting long-term recovery. Collaborative efforts between healthcare providers, policymakers, and communities are essential for improving outcomes for individuals affected by addiction.

9.5. ICD-10 for Substance Use Disorders

This includes several codes for **Substance Use Disorders (SUDs)**, categorized by the type of substance involved and the severity of the disorder (e.g., mild, moderate, or severe).

Each code includes options for conditions with and without associated complications such as withdrawal, dependence, or induced disorders.

1. Alcohol Use Disorder

- **F10.10** – Alcohol abuse, uncomplicated
- **F10.20** – Alcohol dependence, uncomplicated
- **F10.21** – Alcohol dependence, in remission
- **F10.23** – Alcohol dependence with withdrawal
- **F10.24** – Alcohol dependence with alcohol-induced mood disorder

2. Opioid Use Disorder

- **F11.10** – Opioid abuse, uncomplicated
- **F11.20** – Opioid dependence, uncomplicated
- **F11.21** – Opioid dependence, in remission
- **F11.23** – Opioid dependence with withdrawal
- **F11.24** – Opioid dependence with opioid-induced mood disorder

3. Cannabis Use Disorder

- **F12.10** – Cannabis abuse, uncomplicated
- **F12.20** – Cannabis dependence, uncomplicated
- **F12.21** – Cannabis dependence, in remission
- **F12.23** – Cannabis dependence with withdrawal
- **F12.24** – Cannabis dependence with cannabis-induced mood disorder

4. Cocaine Use Disorder

- **F14.10** – Cocaine abuse, uncomplicated
- **F14.20** – Cocaine dependence, uncomplicated
- **F14.21** – Cocaine dependence, in remission
- **F14.23** – Cocaine dependence with withdrawal
- **F14.24** – Cocaine dependence with cocaine-induced mood disorder

5. Sedative, Hypnotic, or Anxiolytic Use Disorder

- **F13.10** – Sedative, hypnotic, or anxiolytic abuse, uncomplicated
- **F13.20** – Sedative, hypnotic, or anxiolytic dependence, uncomplicated
- **F13.21** – Sedative, hypnotic, or anxiolytic dependence, in remission
- **F13.23** – Sedative, hypnotic, or anxiolytic dependence with withdrawal
- **F13.24** – Sedative, hypnotic, or anxiolytic dependence with mood disorder

6. Stimulant Use Disorder (including Amphetamines)

- **F15.10** – Stimulant abuse, uncomplicated
- **F15.20** – Stimulant dependence, uncomplicated
- **F15.21** – Stimulant dependence, in remission
- **F15.23** – Stimulant dependence with withdrawal
- **F15.24** – Stimulant dependence with stimulant-induced mood disorder

7. Hallucinogen Use Disorder

- **F16.10** – Hallucinogen abuse, uncomplicated
- **F16.20** – Hallucinogen dependence, uncomplicated
- **F16.21** – Hallucinogen dependence, in remission
- **F16.24** – Hallucinogen dependence with hallucinogen-induced mood disorder

8. Inhalant Use Disorder

- **F18.10** – Inhalant abuse, uncomplicated
- **F18.20** – Inhalant dependence, uncomplicated
- **F18.21** – Inhalant dependence, in remission
- **F18.24** – Inhalant dependence with inhalant-induced mood disorder

9. Nicotine Dependence

- **F17.200** – Nicotine dependence, unspecified, uncomplicated
- **F17.201** – Nicotine dependence, unspecified, in remission
- **F17.210** – Nicotine dependence, cigarettes, uncomplicated
- **F17.220** – Nicotine dependence, chewing tobacco, uncomplicated

10. Other or Unspecified Substance Use Disorders

- **F19.10** – Other psychoactive substance abuse, uncomplicated
- **F19.20** – Other psychoactive substance dependence, uncomplicated
- **F19.21** – Other psychoactive substance dependence, in remission
- **F19.23** – Other psychoactive substance dependence with withdrawal
- **F19.24** – Other psychoactive substance dependence with substance-induced mood disorder

References:

1. American Psychiatric Association. (2013). *Diagnostic and Statistical Manual of Mental Disorders* (5th ed.).
2. Volkow, N. D., Koob, G. F., & McLellan, A. T. (2016). Neurobiologic advances from the brain disease model of addiction. *New England Journal of Medicine*, 374(4), 363-371.
3. Kranzler, H. R., & Soyka, M. (2018). Diagnosis and pharmacotherapy of alcohol use disorder: A review. *JAMA*, 320(8), 815-824.
4. Soyka, M., Zingg, C., & Koller, G. (2019). Pharmacological treatment of opioid use disorders: A review. *Frontiers in Psychiatry*, 10, 742.
5. McHugh, R. K., & Weiss, R. D. (2019). Alcohol use disorder and co-occurring anxiety, depression, and drug use disorders: A critical review. *Clinical Psychology Review*, 80, 101826.
6. Gowing, L., Farrell, M., Bornemann, R., et al. (2017). Substitution treatment of injecting opioid users for prevention of HIV infection. *Cochrane Database of Systematic Reviews*, 9, CD004145.
7. Barry, C. L., McGinty, E. E., Pescosolido, B. A., & Goldman, H. H. (2014). Stigma, discrimination, treatment effectiveness, and policy: Public views about drug addiction and mental illness. *Psychiatric Services*, 65(10), 1269-1272.

Chapter 10: Eating Disorders

Eating disorders are complex psychiatric conditions characterized by abnormal eating behaviors, distorted body image, and an intense preoccupation with weight and food. They include conditions such as **anorexia nervosa (AN)**, **bulimia nervosa (BN)**, and **binge-eating disorder (BED)**.

These disorders can have severe medical and psychological consequences, making early detection and comprehensive treatment essential. This chapter will explore the characteristics of each major eating disorder, **pharmacotherapy options**, **nutritional interventions**, the importance of an **interdisciplinary approach**, and **supportive care and long-term management strategies**.

10.1. Overview of Anorexia Nervosa, Bulimia Nervosa, and Binge-Eating Disorder

10.1.1. Anorexia Nervosa (AN):

Anorexia nervosa is characterized by **restricted energy intake**, an intense fear of gaining weight, and a distorted body image. Individuals with AN perceive themselves as overweight despite being underweight and engage in extreme behaviors to avoid weight gain, such as excessive dieting, fasting, or compulsive exercise. The DSM-5 diagnostic criteria for anorexia nervosa include:

- **Significantly low body weight** for age, sex, and developmental level.
- **Intense fear of gaining weight** or becoming fat, even though underweight.
- **Disturbance in the perception** of body weight or shape, undue influence of body weight on self-evaluation, or denial of the seriousness of low body weight .

Anorexia is associated with numerous medical complications, including **osteoporosis, cardiac arrhythmias, electrolyte imbalances**, and **amenorrhea**. Individuals with anorexia are at high risk for mortality, both from medical complications and suicide .

10.1.2. Bulimia Nervosa (BN):

Bulimia nervosa involves **recurrent episodes of binge eating** followed by **compensatory behaviors** to prevent weight gain, such as self-induced vomiting, laxative misuse, fasting, or excessive exercise. The binge-purge cycle is driven by extreme concern with body weight and shape, and individuals with BN often maintain a normal weight or are slightly overweight.

The DSM-5 criteria for bulimia nervosa include:

- **Recurrent episodes of binge eating**, defined as consuming an objectively large amount of food in a discrete period (e.g., two hours) and feeling a lack of control over eating.

- **Recurrent inappropriate compensatory behaviors** to prevent weight gain (e.g., vomiting, laxative use).
- Binge eating and compensatory behaviors occur at least **once a week for three months**.
- Self-evaluation is unduly influenced by body shape and weight .

Like AN, bulimia is associated with significant medical complications, such as **electrolyte imbalances**, **esophageal tears**, **dental erosion**, and **cardiac arrhythmias**. Bulimia is also associated with a high risk of comorbid psychiatric disorders, including depression and substance use disorders .

10.1.3. Binge-Eating Disorder (BED):

Binge-eating disorder is characterized by **recurrent episodes of binge eating** without compensatory behaviors such as purging. Individuals with BED experience loss of control over eating and often eat large amounts of food even when not hungry, followed by feelings of guilt, shame, or distress. BED is the most common eating disorder and is often associated with obesity.

The DSM-5 criteria for BED include:

- **Recurrent episodes of binge eating**, defined as eating an unusually large amount of food in a short period and feeling a lack of control.
- Binge episodes are associated with at least three of the following: eating much more rapidly than usual, eating until uncomfortably full, eating large amounts of food when not physically hungry, eating alone due to embarrassment, and feeling disgusted, depressed, or guilty afterward.
- The binge eating occurs, on average, at least **once a week for three months**.
- No regular use of inappropriate compensatory behaviors (e.g., purging) .

10.2. Treatment: Pharmacotherapy Options and Nutritional Interventions

10.2.1. Pharmacotherapy:

Pharmacotherapy plays a supportive role in the treatment of eating disorders, particularly in managing **comorbid psychiatric conditions** like depression, anxiety, or obsessive-compulsive disorder (OCD). While **psychotherapy** and **nutritional rehabilitation** remain the mainstays of treatment, certain medications can help **stabilize mood**, **reduce binge-eating behaviors**, and support **weight gain** in specific eating disorder populations.

1. Anorexia Nervosa (AN)

While no medications are currently **FDA-approved** specifically for the treatment of anorexia nervosa, certain medications may be used off-label to address **comorbid conditions** or support weight gain and mood stabilization.

- **Selective Serotonin Reuptake Inhibitors (SSRIs)**:
  - **SSRIs**, such as **fluoxetine**, are commonly prescribed to treat **comorbid depression** or **anxiety** in individuals with anorexia nervosa, especially after weight stabilization. However, SSRIs alone do not promote weight gain or directly treat the core symptoms of anorexia. Their use is primarily to improve mood and reduce anxiety.
  - **Caution**: SSRIs should be used with caution in patients who are severely malnourished, as their efficacy may be diminished until weight restoration occurs, and they can increase the risk of **QT prolongation**.
- **Olanzapine (atypical antipsychotic)**:
  - **Olanzapine** has been used off-label in anorexia nervosa to promote **weight gain** and help reduce **obsessive thoughts** related to food, weight, and body image. The **antipsychotic** properties of olanzapine help reduce the obsessive-compulsive traits that are often present in patients with anorexia. Additionally, its **appetite-stimulating** effects may contribute to weight restoration.
  - **Evidence**: Some clinical studies have shown modest improvements in **BMI** and **cognitive flexibility** in individuals taking olanzapine, though side effects such as **sedation** and **metabolic changes** must be considered.

2. Bulimia Nervosa (BN)

Pharmacotherapy for bulimia nervosa focuses on reducing **binge-purge cycles** and addressing mood disturbances, particularly **depression** and **anxiety**.

- **Fluoxetine (Prozac)**:
  - **Fluoxetine**, an SSRI, is the **only FDA-approved medication** for the treatment of **bulimia nervosa**. It has been shown to significantly reduce **binge-purge episodes** and improve overall mood in individuals with BN. Unlike its use for depression, higher doses of fluoxetine (typically **60 mg daily**) are often required for therapeutic efficacy in bulimia nervosa.
  - **Mechanism of Action**: Fluoxetine increases **serotonin levels**, which can help regulate mood, reduce anxiety, and decrease impulsivity—key factors in controlling binge-purge behavior.
  - **Other SSRIs**: While fluoxetine is the only FDA-approved SSRI for bulimia, other SSRIs (e.g., **sertraline**, **citalopram**) have also shown efficacy in reducing binge-purge behavior, though they are often used off-label.
- **Topiramate (anticonvulsant)**:
  - **Topiramate** has shown promise in reducing the frequency of **binge-purge episodes** in bulimia nervosa. Although not FDA-approved for BN, it may help decrease **appetite** and reduce **impulsivity** related to binge eating. However, topiramate can cause significant **cognitive side effects** (e.g., memory impairment, difficulty concentrating) and **weight loss**, which can be problematic for individuals with eating disorders.
  - **Caution**: Given its side effect profile, topiramate should be used with caution and close monitoring in individuals with bulimia nervosa.

3. Binge-Eating Disorder (BED)

Binge-eating disorder (BED) is characterized by recurrent episodes of consuming large quantities of food in a short period, accompanied by a sense of **loss of control**. Pharmacotherapy focuses on reducing the frequency of binge-eating episodes and improving **impulse control**.

- **Lisdexamfetamine (Vyvanse)**:
    - **Lisdexamfetamine**, a **stimulant** commonly used to treat **ADHD**, is the only **FDA-approved medication** for the treatment of **binge-eating disorder (BED)**. It works by increasing levels of **dopamine** and **norepinephrine**, which can help regulate **appetite** and reduce **binge-eating episodes**.
    - **Efficacy**: Studies have shown that lisdexamfetamine significantly reduces binge-eating behaviors and improves control over eating. However, because it is a stimulant, it can have side effects such as **insomnia**, **increased heart rate**, and **potential for abuse**, making careful monitoring necessary.
- **Topiramate (anticonvulsant)**:
    - **Topiramate** has also been used off-label to treat BED, primarily by reducing **appetite** and decreasing **binge-eating episodes**. It may be particularly useful for individuals with co-occurring **impulse control** disorders, though its cognitive side effects and weight loss potential need to be considered, especially in patients with BED who may already struggle with **body image issues**.
- **SSRIs (Selective Serotonin Reuptake Inhibitors)**:
    - **SSRIs**, such as **fluoxetine** and **sertraline**, are commonly used off-label for the treatment of **BED**, especially in patients with comorbid **depression** or **anxiety**. While not FDA-approved specifically for BED, SSRIs can help reduce binge-eating episodes by stabilizing mood and decreasing **compulsive eating behaviors**.

10.2.2. Nutritional Interventions:

Nutritional rehabilitation is a critical component in the treatment of eating disorders, serving as a foundation for physical recovery and psychological healing. Each eating disorder presents unique nutritional challenges, with malnutrition often having severe consequences on the body's physiological systems.

The primary goals of nutritional interventions are to restore **healthy weight**, **normalize eating patterns**, and address the **medical complications** that arise from **poor nutrition**.

1. Anorexia Nervosa (AN)

In **anorexia nervosa**, patients experience extreme **caloric restriction** and significant **weight loss**, which often results in severe **malnutrition**. Nutritional interventions in AN are designed to gradually restore a **healthy body weight**, correct **nutritional deficiencies**, and ensure safe refeeding practices to avoid complications like **refeeding syndrome**.

- **Structured Meal Plans**:
    - Individuals with AN require highly structured meal plans to **increase caloric intake** gradually and consistently. Meal plans are often developed by **registered dietitians** in collaboration with the treatment team, aiming to restore weight at a safe and controlled rate (typically **1–3 pounds per week** for hospitalized patients, and **0.5–1 pound per week** in outpatient settings).
    - Meal plans should be nutritionally balanced, emphasizing a wide variety of **macronutrients** (carbohydrates, proteins, and fats) and **micronutrients** (vitamins and minerals) to ensure **full nutritional recovery**. **Caloric density** is often increased over time as the patient's body adjusts to eating larger amounts of food.
- **Enteral Feeding and Hospitalization**:
    - In severe cases of AN, where patients are at **high risk of medical complications** or refuse to eat, **hospitalization** and **enteral feeding** (tube feeding) may be necessary. Enteral feeding can provide the **necessary calories** and nutrients for patients who are unable or unwilling to consume adequate food orally.
    - **Parenteral nutrition** (intravenous feeding) is rarely used, but may be considered in critically ill patients with **gastrointestinal dysfunction**.
- **Monitoring for Refeeding Syndrome**:
    - **Refeeding syndrome** is a potentially fatal complication that can occur when malnourished individuals are **refed too rapidly**. It involves a dangerous shift in **electrolytes** (primarily **phosphate**, **potassium**, and **magnesium**) and fluids, which can lead to **cardiac, respiratory, and neurological complications**.
    - To prevent refeeding syndrome, caloric intake is increased **gradually**, and electrolyte levels (especially **phosphorus**) are closely monitored during the refeeding process. Supplementation of **electrolytes**, **thiamine**, and **multivitamins** is often initiated at the start of refeeding to reduce the risk of complications.
- **Addressing Psychological Resistance to Weight Gain**:
    - Individuals with AN often experience **intense fear** of weight gain and **distorted body image**, making nutritional rehabilitation particularly challenging. **Therapeutic support** is integrated with nutritional interventions to address the **psychological resistance** to eating and gaining weight. **Cognitive behavioral therapy (CBT)** is often used in conjunction with meal plans to help patients challenge their fears and misconceptions about food and weight.

2. Bulimia Nervosa (BN) and Binge-Eating Disorder (BED)

In **bulimia nervosa** and **binge-eating disorder**, the focus of nutritional counseling is to **break the cycles** of **binge eating** and **purging** (in BN) or **compulsive overeating** (in BED). Nutritional interventions aim to establish **regular eating patterns**, prevent **deprivation**, and stabilize **blood sugar levels**, which can help reduce binge-eating episodes and improve overall nutritional status.

- **Regular, Balanced Meals**:
    - In both BN and BED, the goal is to develop **structured eating patterns** with **regular meals** and snacks throughout the day to prevent the **cycle of deprivation** that often leads to **binge eating**. Dietitians work closely with patients to create **meal plans** that are nutritionally balanced and provide **adequate caloric intake** without **restrictive dieting**.
    - Encouraging **consistent eating** (e.g., three meals and two snacks daily) helps stabilize **blood sugar levels** and reduces the urge to binge. Structured meal plans also prevent **unhealthy compensatory behaviors** such as **purging**, **excessive exercise**, or **fasting** after eating.
- **Eliminating Binge-Purge Cycles** (for BN):
    - Nutritional interventions for BN focus on **eliminating binge-purge episodes** by addressing the **restrict-binge-purge cycle**. Often, patients restrict their intake during the day, which leads to **overeating** or **bingeing** later. Establishing regular, planned meals helps prevent hunger-driven binge eating.
    - Patients are educated on **normalizing eating behaviors**, managing **hunger cues**, and avoiding **trigger foods** that may lead to binge episodes. Dietitians provide support in helping individuals eat **balanced meals** that include all food groups, which helps reduce the psychological and physiological triggers for binge-purge episodes.
- **Nutritional Rehabilitation in BED**:
    - For patients with **binge-eating disorder**, nutritional interventions focus on reducing **compulsive overeating** and improving **portion control**. This includes addressing **emotional triggers** for overeating and working with patients to develop **healthy eating habits** that promote satiety and satisfaction without relying on food as a coping mechanism.
    - **Mindful eating techniques** may also be introduced to help patients slow down their eating, recognize **hunger and fullness cues**, and enjoy food in a healthy, balanced manner.
- **Addressing Nutrient Deficiencies and Electrolyte Imbalances**:
    - In both BN and BED, **electrolyte imbalances** (particularly **hypokalemia**) can occur as a result of **purging** or excessive **laxative use**. Nutritional interventions include **correcting electrolyte deficiencies** and educating patients on the dangers of **purging behaviors**.
    - Patients with BED may also have **nutritional deficiencies** due to **poor diet quality**, particularly if binge eating involves **high-calorie, low-nutrient foods**. Dietitians work to improve the overall quality of the diet, ensuring that patients receive adequate **vitamins** and **minerals** through their meals.

10.3. Interdisciplinary Approach to Treating Eating Disorders

Eating disorders are multifaceted, requiring a comprehensive, interdisciplinary approach involving medical, nutritional, and psychological care. Effective treatment often involves a combination of the following professionals:

- **Physicians**: Medical professionals are essential for managing the physical health consequences of eating disorders, such as malnutrition, electrolyte imbalances, and cardiac complications. Regular monitoring of weight, vital signs, and laboratory values is necessary to detect and address complications.
- **Dietitians**: Dietitians play a key role in nutritional rehabilitation, developing meal plans that promote weight restoration in AN and normalizing eating behaviors in BN and BED. They educate patients about healthy eating patterns and help address food-related anxieties.
- **Mental Health Professionals**: Psychiatrists, psychologists, and therapists provide psychotherapy, which is the mainstay of treatment for eating disorders. **Cognitive Behavioral Therapy (CBT)**, especially **CBT-E** (enhanced CBT for eating disorders), is considered the gold standard for treating BN and BED, and has been adapted for use in AN. **Family-Based Treatment (FBT)**, also known as the **Maudsley Method**, is often used for adolescents with AN and involves the entire family in supporting the individual's recovery .

10.4. Supportive Care and Long-Term Management Strategies

10.4.1. Supportive Care:

Supportive care is critical to managing the medical, psychological, and social aspects of eating disorders. Treatment often requires a long-term commitment and relapse prevention strategies.

- **Psychotherapy**: In addition to CBT and FBT, other psychotherapies such as **Dialectical Behavior Therapy (DBT)** and **Interpersonal Therapy (IPT)** may be used to address underlying emotional and relational issues. DBT is particularly helpful in managing emotional dysregulation, which is common in eating disorders.
- **Monitoring and Medical Management**: Continuous monitoring of physical health is essential, particularly in individuals with AN who are at risk for life-threatening medical complications. Regular follow-up visits with medical professionals help ensure that weight and health parameters remain stable.

10.4.2. Long-Term Management and Relapse Prevention:

Eating disorders often require long-term management due to their chronic nature and high relapse rates. Strategies to promote long-term recovery include:

- **Building Resilience**: Patients are encouraged to build coping skills to manage stress, anxiety, and emotions without resorting to disordered eating behaviors. This can involve

learning **mindfulness techniques, emotion regulation,** and **problem-solving strategies**.
- **Social Support**: Support from family, friends, and peer groups is crucial for maintaining recovery. Participation in **support groups**, such as those offered by the **National Eating Disorders Association (NEDA)**, can provide ongoing encouragement and a sense of community .
- **Addressing Comorbid Conditions**: Many individuals with eating disorders also suffer from comorbid psychiatric conditions, such as depression, anxiety, OCD, or substance use disorders. Integrated treatment addressing both the eating disorder and any co-occurring conditions is necessary for sustained recovery.

Eating disorders are serious psychiatric conditions with significant physical, emotional, and social consequences. A comprehensive treatment plan involving pharmacotherapy, nutritional rehabilitation, psychotherapy, and medical monitoring is essential for successful management. An interdisciplinary approach that includes physicians, dietitians, and mental health professionals provides the best chance for recovery. Long-term management and relapse prevention require ongoing support, addressing both the psychological and physical aspects of the disorder.

10.5. ICD-10 for eating disorders

These codes cover the primary eating disorders as well as less specific or other eating-related conditions. Accurate coding is important for diagnosis, treatment, and insurance purposes.

Anorexia Nervosa

- **F50.00** – Anorexia nervosa, unspecified
- **F50.01** – Anorexia nervosa, restricting type
- **F50.02** – Anorexia nervosa, binge-eating/purging type

Bulimia Nervosa

- **F50.2** – Bulimia nervosa

Binge-Eating Disorder (BED)

- **F50.81** – Binge-eating disorder

Other Eating Disorders

- **F50.89** – Other specified eating disorder (e.g., atypical anorexia nervosa, night eating syndrome)
- **F50.9** – Eating disorder, unspecified

References:

1. American Psychiatric Association. (2013). *Diagnostic and Statistical Manual of Mental Disorders* (5th ed.).
2. Kaye, W. H., Wierenga, C. E., Bailer, U. F., et al. (2013). Nothing tastes as good as skinny feels: The neurobiology of anorexia nervosa. *Trends in Neurosciences*, 36(2), 110-120.
3. Keel, P. K., & Brown, T. A. (2010). Update on course and outcome in eating disorders. *International Journal of Eating Disorders*, 43(3), 195-204.
4. Mitchell, J. E., & Peterson, C. B. (2020). Anorexia nervosa. *New England Journal of Medicine*, 382(14), 1343-1351.
5. Bulik, C. M., Brownley, K. A., Shapiro, J. R., et al. (2010). Binge-eating disorder: A comprehensive review. *International Journal of Eating Disorders*, 43(5), 361-370.
6. Hay, P., Claudino, A. M., Touyz, S., & Abd Elbaky, G. (2015). Individual psychological therapy in the outpatient treatment of adults with anorexia nervosa. *Cochrane Database of Systematic Reviews*, 7, CD003909.
7. Treasure, J., Stein, D., & Maguire, S. (2015). Has the time come to classify eating disorders on the basis of neurobiology? *BMC Medicine*, 13, 72.

Chapter 11: Sleep-Wake Disorders

Sleep-wake disorders encompass a range of conditions that affect the quality, timing, and amount of sleep, leading to significant distress or impaired daytime functioning. Common sleep-wake disorders include **insomnia**, **hypersomnia**, **circadian rhythm sleep-wake disorders**, **sleep apnea**, **parasomnias**, **Restless Legs Syndrome (RLS)**, and **narcolepsy**.

This chapter will provide an overview of these disorders, explore **pharmacotherapy options** (including sedative-hypnotics, melatonin agonists, and orexin receptor antagonists), and discuss **behavioral interventions** such as sleep hygiene, as well as methods for **monitoring and optimizing pharmacotherapy**.

11.1. Overview of Sleep-Wake Disorders

11.1.1. Insomnia Disorder

Insomnia is characterized by persistent difficulty with sleep initiation, duration, consolidation, or quality despite adequate opportunities to sleep, leading to daytime impairment.

DSM-5 Diagnostic Criteria:

- **A.** A predominant complaint of dissatisfaction with sleep quantity or quality, associated with one (or more) of the following symptoms:
    - Difficulty initiating sleep
    - Difficulty maintaining sleep (e.g., frequent awakenings or trouble returning to sleep after awakenings)
    - Early-morning awakening with an inability to return to sleep
- **B.** The sleep disturbance causes clinically significant distress or impairment in social, occupational, educational, academic, behavioral, or other important areas of functioning.
- **C.** The sleep difficulty occurs at least **3 nights per week**.
- **D.** The sleep difficulty is present for at least **3 months**.
- **E.** The sleep difficulty occurs despite adequate opportunity for sleep.

Symptoms:

- Difficulty falling asleep, staying asleep, or waking up too early
- Daytime fatigue, irritability, and difficulty concentrating

Treatment:

- **Cognitive-behavioral therapy for insomnia (CBT-I)**
- **Pharmacotherapy**: Short-term use of sedative-hypnotics (e.g., benzodiazepines, Z-drugs), melatonin agonists, or orexin receptor antagonists

- **Sleep hygiene**: Regular sleep schedule, avoiding caffeine before bed, and creating a comfortable sleep environment

11.1.2. Hypersomnolence Disorder (Hypersomnia)

Hypersomnolence disorder involves excessive daytime sleepiness despite sufficient sleep duration during the night, with a strong urge to sleep or prolonged sleep episodes during the day.

DSM-5 Diagnostic Criteria:

- **A.** Self-reported excessive sleepiness (hypersomnolence) despite a main sleep period lasting at least **7 hours**, with at least one of the following:
    - Recurrent periods of sleep or lapses into sleep within the same day
    - A prolonged main sleep episode of more than **9 hours** per day that is non-restorative (i.e., unrefreshing)
    - Difficulty being fully awake after abrupt awakening
- **B.** The hypersomnolence occurs at least **3 times per week**, for at least **3 months**.
- **C.** The hypersomnolence causes clinically significant distress or impairment in social, occupational, or other important areas of functioning.

Symptoms:

- Excessive daytime sleepiness, despite long sleep periods
- Difficulty waking up in the morning
- Cognitive impairment and memory problems during the day

Treatment:

- **Stimulants** (e.g., modafinil, amphetamines)
- **Scheduled naps** and improvement of sleep hygiene

11.1.3. Circadian Rhythm Sleep-Wake Disorders

Circadian rhythm disorders are characterized by a misalignment between the individual's internal biological clock and the external environment, resulting in disrupted sleep patterns and impaired functioning.

DSM-5 Diagnostic Criteria:

- **A.** A persistent or recurrent pattern of sleep disruption that is primarily due to an alteration of the circadian system or a misalignment between the endogenous circadian rhythm and the sleep-wake schedule required by an individual's physical environment or social or professional schedule.
- **B.** The sleep disruption leads to excessive sleepiness or insomnia, or both.

- **C.** The sleep disturbance causes clinically significant distress or impairment in social, occupational, and other important areas of functioning.

Types:

- **Delayed Sleep Phase Disorder**: Difficulty falling asleep and waking up at conventional times.
- **Advanced Sleep Phase Disorder**: Falling asleep and waking up earlier than desired.
- **Irregular Sleep-Wake Rhythm**: Fragmented sleep patterns with no consistent pattern.
- **Shift Work Disorder**: Difficulty adjusting to work schedules outside the typical 9-to-5 structure (e.g., night shifts).
- **Jet Lag**: Temporary sleep-wake cycle disruption due to crossing time zones.

Treatment:

- **Light therapy** to reset circadian rhythms
- **Melatonin supplements** or **melatonin agonists** for sleep onset issues
- **Chronotherapy**: Gradually adjusting sleep times to realign the circadian rhythm

11.1.4. Obstructive Sleep Apnea Hypopnea

Sleep apnea is a condition in which breathing repeatedly stops and starts during sleep, disrupting normal sleep cycles. The most common type is **obstructive sleep apnea (OSA)**, where the airway is blocked during sleep.

DSM-5 Diagnostic Criteria:

- **A.** Either (1) or (2):
  - (1) **Evidence** by polysomnography of at least **five obstructive apneas** or hypopneas per hour of sleep and either of the following symptoms:
    - Nocturnal breathing disturbances (e.g., snoring, gasping, breathing pauses)
    - Daytime sleepiness, fatigue, or unrefreshing sleep despite sufficient opportunities to sleep
  - (2) Evidence by polysomnography of **15 or more obstructive apneas** and/or hypopneas per hour of sleep, regardless of accompanying symptoms.

Symptoms:

- Loud snoring, gasping for air during sleep
- Episodes of breathing cessation during sleep
- Daytime fatigue and poor concentration
- Morning headaches

Treatment:

- **Continuous Positive Airway Pressure (CPAP)** device to keep the airway open during sleep
- **Weight loss** and lifestyle modifications
- **Surgery** for severe cases of airway obstruction

11.1.5. Parasomnias

Parasomnias are abnormal behaviors or experiences that occur during sleep or sleep transitions, including sleepwalking, night terrors, and REM sleep behavior disorder.

DSM-5 Diagnostic Criteria for Non-REM Sleep Arousal Disorders (e.g., sleepwalking, night terrors):

- **A.** Recurrent episodes of incomplete awakening from sleep, usually occurring during the first third of the major sleep episode, accompanied by either sleepwalking or sleep terrors.
- **B.** No or little dream imagery is recalled.
- **C.** Amnesia for the episodes is present.
- **D.** The episodes cause significant distress or impairment in functioning.

Symptoms:

- **Sleepwalking**: Engaging in complex behaviors while still asleep, with no memory of the event.
- **Night terrors**: Waking abruptly in a terrified state, often with screaming or thrashing, with no memory of the episode.
- **REM Sleep Behavior Disorder**: Acting out vivid dreams during REM sleep, often involving violent or dangerous behaviors.

Treatment:

- **Safety measures** to prevent injury during episodes
- **Medications** such as **benzodiazepines** or **melatonin** for REM sleep behavior disorder

11.1.6. Restless Legs Syndrome (RLS)

Restless Legs Syndrome is a neurological disorder characterized by uncomfortable sensations in the legs, accompanied by an irresistible urge to move them, especially during periods of rest.

DSM-5 Diagnostic Criteria:

- **A.** An urge to move the legs, usually accompanied by or in response to uncomfortable and unpleasant sensations in the legs, characterized by all of the following:
    - The urge to move the legs begins or worsens during periods of rest or inactivity.
    - The urge to move the legs is partially or totally relieved by movement.

- The urge to move the legs is worse in the evening or at night than during the day, or occurs only in the evening or night.
- **B.** The symptoms occur at least **3 times per week**, persist for at least **3 months**, and cause significant distress or impairment in functioning.

Symptoms:

- Uncomfortable leg sensations (e.g., tingling, burning) that are relieved by movement
- Difficulty falling or staying asleep due to discomfort
- Daytime fatigue from disrupted sleep

Treatment:

- **Dopaminergic agents** (e.g., pramipexole, ropinirole)
- **Iron supplementation** (if low ferritin levels)
- **Lifestyle modifications** such as regular exercise and avoiding caffeine

11.1.7. Narcolepsy

Narcolepsy is a chronic neurological disorder characterized by excessive daytime sleepiness and sudden, uncontrollable episodes of falling asleep. It often includes **cataplexy**, a sudden loss of muscle tone triggered by strong emotions.

DSM-5 Diagnostic Criteria:

- **A.** Recurrent periods of an irrepressible need to sleep, lapsing into sleep, or napping occurring within the same day. These must have been occurring at least **3 times per week** over the past **3 months**.
- **B.** The presence of at least one of the following:
  - Episodes of **cataplexy** occurring at least a few times per month.
  - **Hypocretin deficiency**, measured via cerebrospinal fluid.
  - Nocturnal sleep polysomnography showing REM sleep latency of **15 minutes or less**, or a mean sleep latency of **8 minutes or less** on a Multiple Sleep Latency Test (MSLT).

Symptoms:

- Sudden, overwhelming daytime sleepiness
- Cataplexy (sudden muscle weakness triggered by emotions)
- **Sleep paralysis** (temporary inability to move upon waking)
- **Hypnagogic hallucinations** (vivid dream-like experiences while falling asleep)

Treatment:

- **Stimulants** (e.g., modafinil, amphetamines) for daytime sleepiness
- **Sodium oxybate** for cataplexy and improving sleep quality

- **Antidepressants** for managing cataplexy

11.2. Pharmacotherapy Options: Sedative-Hypnotics, Melatonin Agonists, and Orexin Receptor Antagonists

Pharmacotherapy is a critical option for managing **insomnia** when behavioral interventions alone are insufficient. Several classes of medications are available, each with unique mechanisms of action, benefits, and potential risks. These include **sedative-hypnotics**, **melatonin agonists**, and **orexin receptor antagonists**, all of which aim to improve sleep quality and duration in different ways.

11.2.1. Sedative-Hypnotics

Sedative-hypnotics are a commonly used group of medications that act by enhancing **inhibitory neurotransmission** in the central nervous system, primarily through their action on **GABA-A receptors**, which facilitate sleep.

- **Benzodiazepines**:
    - **Benzodiazepines** like **temazepam** and **lorazepam** are among the most established sedative-hypnotics. These medications promote sleep by enhancing the activity of **gamma-aminobutyric acid (GABA)**, the brain's main inhibitory neurotransmitter. By binding to the **GABA-A receptor**, they reduce **sleep latency** (the time it takes to fall asleep) and **increase total sleep time**.
    - **Limitations**: Despite their efficacy, benzodiazepines are associated with several significant drawbacks, including the development of **tolerance**, **dependence**, and **rebound insomnia** when the medication is discontinued. Long-term use can also result in **cognitive side effects** such as **memory impairment** and **daytime sedation**. Because of these risks, benzodiazepines are recommended primarily for **short-term management of insomnia**.
    - **Examples**:
        - **Temazepam**: Commonly used for short-term relief of insomnia due to its intermediate duration of action.
        - **Lorazepam**: Often used in acute settings but also recommended for short durations.
- **Non-Benzodiazepine Sedative-Hypnotics (Z-Drugs)**:
    - **Z-drugs**, including **zolpidem (Ambien)**, **zaleplon (Sonata)**, and **eszopiclone (Lunesta)**, are also **GABA-A receptor agonists**, but they have a more selective action on the **alpha-1 subunit** of the receptor, which is specifically linked to sedation.
    - **Benefits**: Due to their **selectivity**, Z-drugs are associated with **fewer side effects** than traditional benzodiazepines, such as less **daytime sedation** and a **lower risk of dependence**. They are also less likely to impair cognitive function, making them suitable for **longer-term use** in some cases, although regular revaluation is recommended.
    - **Examples**:

- **Zolpidem (Ambien)**: Effective for both sleep onset and maintenance insomnia, but should be used with caution due to potential for next-day drowsiness.
- **Eszopiclone (Lunesta)**: Particularly effective for **sleep maintenance**, with studies showing it can be used safely over extended periods for chronic insomnia.
  - **Risks**: Z-drugs, while considered safer than benzodiazepines, can still carry a risk of **abuse** and **dependence** with prolonged use. Rare side effects like **sleepwalking** or **complex sleep behaviors** (e.g., eating, driving while not fully awake) have been reported, particularly with zolpidem.

11.2.2. Melatonin Agonists

Melatonin is a natural hormone produced by the **pineal gland** that regulates the body's **circadian rhythms** and **sleep-wake cycles**. **Melatonin agonists**, which mimic the action of endogenous melatonin, are particularly useful for **circadian rhythm disorders** and **sleep-onset insomnia**.

- **Melatonin Supplements**:
  - **Exogenous melatonin supplements** are commonly used for short-term management of insomnia, especially in individuals with **jet lag**, **shift work disorder**, or **delayed sleep phase syndrome**. While over-the-counter melatonin supplements can be beneficial in realigning the circadian rhythm, they have limited efficacy in managing **chronic insomnia**.
- **Ramelteon (Rozerem)**:
  - **Ramelteon** is a **melatonin receptor agonist** and the only **FDA-approved** medication of its kind for the treatment of **sleep-onset insomnia**. Ramelteon works by selectively binding to **MT1** and **MT2** receptors in the brain, which are critical for regulating circadian rhythms and promoting the onset of sleep.
  - **Benefits**: Unlike sedative-hypnotics, **ramelteon** does not act on **GABA** pathways, making it **non-addictive** and associated with a **lower risk of dependence** or **withdrawal symptoms**. It is particularly useful for **older adults** and those with sleep disorders related to **circadian rhythm disturbances**.
  - **Applications**: Ramelteon is especially helpful in populations that may not tolerate traditional hypnotics, such as the **elderly** or patients with a history of **substance abuse**, since it has a favorable safety profile and minimal risk for **next-day sedation**.

11.2.3. Orexin Receptor Antagonists

The **orexin system** plays a central role in **wakefulness** by promoting **arousal** and **alertness**. **Orexin receptor antagonists** are a newer class of drugs that work by blocking the action of **orexin** to promote **sleep**. They offer a novel mechanism of action compared to traditional sedative-hypnotics.

- **Suvorexant (Belsomra)**:
  - **Suvorexant** is the first **FDA-approved orexin receptor antagonist**, effective for both **sleep-onset** and **sleep-maintenance insomnia**. It works by blocking **orexin A** and **orexin B** receptors, which reduces wakefulness, allowing for the initiation and maintenance of sleep.
  - **Benefits**: Unlike benzodiazepines or Z-drugs, suvorexant does not directly sedate the patient. Instead, it helps to suppress **wakefulness** without affecting other neurotransmitter systems, leading to a **lower risk of dependence** and **minimal cognitive side effects**.
  - **Side Effects**: **Suvorexant** is generally well tolerated, but side effects can include **daytime drowsiness**, **unusual dreams**, and in some cases, **sleep paralysis** or **hypnagogic hallucinations**. It may also impair **driving ability** the next morning, particularly at higher doses.
- **Lemborexant**:
  - **Lemborexant**, another **orexin receptor antagonist**, is used to treat **insomnia** characterized by difficulty with sleep onset and maintenance. Studies have shown it is effective in improving both sleep duration and quality with a favorable safety profile.
  - **Advantages**: Like suvorexant, lemborexant is associated with **lower abuse potential** compared to sedative-hypnotics, making it a safer option for long-term use in chronic insomnia.

11.3. Behavioral Interventions and Sleep Hygiene Recommendations

Cognitive Behavioral Therapy for Insomnia (CBT-I) is the first-line treatment for chronic insomnia, with strong evidence supporting its effectiveness. It combines cognitive and behavioral techniques to address the underlying thoughts and behaviors contributing to insomnia.

11.3.1. Cognitive Behavioral Therapy for Insomnia (CBT-I):

CBT-I involves several components aimed at improving sleep quality and reducing sleep-related anxiety:

- **Cognitive restructuring**: Identifying and challenging unhelpful beliefs about sleep (e.g., "I need eight hours of sleep every night to function").
- **Stimulus control**: Encouraging behaviors that promote sleep (e.g., going to bed only when sleepy, getting out of bed if unable to sleep) and eliminating behaviors that disrupt sleep (e.g., watching TV in bed).
- **Sleep restriction**: Limiting time in bed to increase sleep drive and reduce the frustration of being unable to sleep.
- **Relaxation techniques**: Using deep breathing, progressive muscle relaxation, or mindfulness to reduce physiological arousal before bedtime.

11.3.2. Sleep Hygiene:

Good sleep hygiene is essential for optimizing sleep quality. Recommendations include:

- **Maintaining a regular sleep schedule**: Going to bed and waking up at the same time every day, even on weekends.
- **Creating a restful sleep environment**: Keeping the bedroom dark, quiet, and cool, and using a comfortable mattress and pillow.
- **Avoiding stimulants**: Limiting caffeine, nicotine, and heavy meals close to bedtime.
- **Limiting screen time**: Reducing exposure to blue light from phones, computers, and TVs before bed, as it can interfere with melatonin production.
- **Engaging in regular physical activity**: Exercise during the day promotes better sleep, but vigorous exercise close to bedtime should be avoided.

11.4. Monitoring and Optimizing Pharmacotherapy for Sleep Disorders

Effective management of **sleep disorders** requires not only the appropriate selection of pharmacotherapy but also regular **monitoring**, **optimization**, and integration of **behavioral interventions**. The goal is to maximize treatment benefits while minimizing risks, particularly for long-term use.

11.4.1. Monitoring Efficacy and Side Effects

Pharmacotherapy for sleep disorders must be closely monitored to evaluate its **effectiveness** and identify any **adverse effects**. This process involves regular follow-up appointments to assess the patient's response to the medication and make necessary adjustments.

- **Efficacy Monitoring**:
    - Patients should be asked about improvements in their **sleep quality**, including changes in **sleep latency** (the time it takes to fall asleep), **sleep duration**, and **sleep maintenance** (ability to stay asleep without frequent awakenings). **Sleep diaries** or **sleep trackers** can help document these changes more objectively.
    - **Patient-reported outcomes** should be regularly reviewed, including how well they feel rested during the day, whether they experience **daytime fatigue**, and any impact on their **overall functioning**.
- **Monitoring for Side Effects**:
    - **Daytime drowsiness**, **cognitive impairment**, and **falls**, particularly in **older adults**, are common side effects of sedative-hypnotic medications. Older patients are at increased risk of **falls** and **fractures** due to sedation and impaired motor coordination. This risk is further heightened by polypharmacy, where multiple medications can interact to increase sedative effects.
    - **Dependence and tolerance** are concerns with **benzodiazepines** and **Z-drugs**. Patients should be educated about the **risk of dependence** and the possibility of **rebound insomnia** when these medications are discontinued abruptly.
    - Patients should also be informed about **uncommon but serious side effects**, such as **complex sleep behaviors** (e.g., sleepwalking, sleep-driving), which can occur with non-benzodiazepine sedative-hypnotics (e.g., zolpidem).

- **Periodic Reassessment**:
    - It is critical to regularly reassess whether the patient continues to benefit from the medication or if they can transition to **non-pharmacological treatments**. For instance, medications like **benzodiazepines** should be used cautiously and for short durations due to risks associated with **long-term use**.
    - For patients on long-term therapy, reevaluation should include assessing any signs of **tolerance** or **dependence**, and considering whether **discontinuation** or **tapering** might be appropriate.

11.4.2. Addressing Long-Term Use and Tapering

While sleep medications such as **benzodiazepines** and **Z-drugs** are effective for **short-term use**, they are not always recommended for long-term management due to the risks of **tolerance, dependence,** and **withdrawal symptoms**. Careful management is required when discontinuing these medications.

- **Risks of Long-Term Use**:
    - **Benzodiazepines** and non-benzodiazepine sedative-hypnotics, such as **zolpidem** or **eszopiclone**, carry a high risk of **tolerance** over time, meaning patients may require higher doses to achieve the same therapeutic effect. This can also lead to **dependence**, where the body becomes reliant on the medication to initiate sleep.
    - Long-term use can result in **withdrawal symptoms** (e.g., **rebound insomnia, anxiety, agitation**) when the medication is discontinued abruptly. In severe cases, particularly with **benzodiazepines**, withdrawal can cause **seizures** or **delirium**.
- **Tapering Protocol**:
    - To prevent withdrawal symptoms and rebound insomnia, it is recommended to **gradually taper** sleep medications, especially in patients who have been using them for an extended period. A typical tapering schedule involves **reducing the dose** by a small percentage (e.g., 10-25%) every **1-2 weeks**, depending on the medication and the patient's tolerance.
    - Close **monitoring** during the tapering process is essential to adjust the tapering speed based on how well the patient tolerates dose reductions. In some cases, switching from a **short-acting benzodiazepine** to a **longer-acting agent** (such as **diazepam**) may help ease the tapering process by providing more stable blood levels.
- **Management of Withdrawal and Rebound Insomnia**:
    - Patients discontinuing sedative-hypnotics may experience **rebound insomnia** (temporary worsening of sleep difficulties), which can last for a few days to a week. To manage this, behavioral strategies like **sleep hygiene education** and **cognitive-behavioral therapy for insomnia (CBT-I)** can be helpful in mitigating symptoms.
    - **Adjunctive medications** (e.g., **melatonin agonists** or **antidepressants**) may sometimes be used temporarily to ease the transition during tapering.

11.4.3. Combination of Pharmacotherapy and Behavioral Interventions

For patients with **chronic insomnia**, combining **pharmacotherapy** with **behavioral interventions** offers a more comprehensive approach to treatment. **Cognitive-behavioral therapy for insomnia (CBT-I)** is widely recognized as the gold standard for long-term insomnia management and is often more effective when combined with medications for short-term symptom relief.

- **Cognitive-Behavioral Therapy for Insomnia (CBT-I)**:
    - **CBT-I** focuses on modifying behaviors and thoughts that contribute to chronic insomnia. It includes strategies such as **stimulus control**, **sleep restriction**, **cognitive restructuring**, and **sleep hygiene education**. Patients learn how to **reframe negative thoughts** about sleep and develop healthy sleep habits that promote long-term sleep quality.
    - **Studies show** that combining **CBT-I** with pharmacotherapy can result in faster improvements in sleep quality compared to either treatment alone, particularly during the initial phase of treatment. Over time, as patients improve their sleep behaviors and routines, they may be able to **reduce** or **discontinue** their medication.
- **Pharmacotherapy as a Bridge**:
    - Medications can provide **short-term relief** while patients work on implementing behavioral changes through **CBT-I**. For example, a patient with severe sleep onset insomnia may start with **zolpidem** for immediate symptom relief while engaging in **behavioral therapy** to address underlying sleep issues.
    - Over time, as patients become more comfortable with new sleep habits, medications can often be **tapered** or discontinued under medical supervision.
- **Follow-Up and Support**:
    - Long-term success in treating sleep disorders often depends on **regular follow-up** and ongoing **support** from healthcare providers. Continuous assessment of the patient's progress with **behavioral therapy** and **sleep medications** is critical to determining whether further adjustments are necessary.
    - Patients should be educated about the **importance of adherence** to both behavioral and pharmacological treatment components, as well as how to manage occasional setbacks.

11.5. ICD-10 for Sleep-wake Disorders

These ICD-10 codes cover a range of sleep-wake disorders, including insomnia, hypersomnia, circadian rhythm disorders, sleep apnea, parasomnias, and narcolepsy. Accurate coding is important for diagnosis, treatment, and reimbursement in clinical settings.

Insomnia Disorders

- **G47.00** – Insomnia, unspecified
- **F51.01** – Primary insomnia (nonorganic origin)

- **F51.09** – Other insomnia (nonorganic origin)

Hypersomnia Disorders

- **G47.10** – Hypersomnia, unspecified
- **F51.11** – Primary hypersomnia
- **F51.12** – Nonorganic hypersomnia

Circadian Rhythm Sleep-Wake Disorders

- **G47.20** – Circadian rhythm sleep disorder, unspecified type
- **G47.21** – Circadian rhythm sleep disorder, delayed sleep phase type
- **G47.22** – Circadian rhythm sleep disorder, advanced sleep phase type
- **G47.23** – Circadian rhythm sleep disorder, irregular sleep-wake type
- **G47.24** – Circadian rhythm sleep disorder, free-running type
- **G47.26** – Circadian rhythm sleep disorder, shift work type

Sleep Apnea Disorders

- **G47.30** – Sleep apnea, unspecified
- **G47.33** – Obstructive sleep apnea (adult) (pediatric)
- **G47.31** – Central sleep apnea
- **G47.32** – Complex sleep apnea syndrome (treatment-emergent central sleep apnea)

Parasomnias

- **G47.50** – Parasomnia, unspecified
- **G47.51** – REM sleep behavior disorder
- **G47.52** – Sleepwalking (somnambulism)
- **G47.53** – Sleep terrors (night terrors)
- **G47.54** – Sleep paralysis

Restless Legs Syndrome

- **G25.81** – Restless legs syndrome

Narcolepsy and Cataplexy

- **G47.411** – Narcolepsy with cataplexy
- **G47.419** – Narcolepsy without cataplexy
- **G47.42** – Narcolepsy in conditions classified elsewhere

References:

1. American Academy of Sleep Medicine. (2014). *International Classification of Sleep Disorders* (3rd ed.).

2. American Psychiatric Association. (2013). *Diagnostic and Statistical Manual of Mental Disorders* (5th ed.).
3. Riemann, D., Baglioni, C., Bassetti, C., et al. (2017). European guideline for the diagnosis and treatment of insomnia. *Journal of Sleep Research*, 26(6), 675-700.
4. Winkelman, J. W. (2015). Insomnia disorder. *New England Journal of Medicine*, 373(15), 1437-1444.
5. Krystal, A. D. (2019). Pharmacological treatment of insomnia. *Advances in Pharmacology*, 84, 241-253.
6. Schwartz, J. R., & Roth, T. (2008). Neurophysiology of sleep and wakefulness: Basic science and clinical implications. *Current Neuropharmacology*, 6(4), 367-378.
7. Qaseem, A., Kansagara, D., Forciea, M. A., et al. (2016). Management of chronic insomnia disorder in adults: A clinical practice guideline from the American College of Physicians. *Annals of Internal Medicine*, 165(2), 125-133.

Chapter 12: Personality Disorders

Personality disorders are a group of mental health conditions characterized by enduring, inflexible, and maladaptive patterns of thinking, feeling, behaving, and relating to others. These patterns deviate markedly from societal expectations, impair daily functioning, and cause distress to the individual or those around them. Managing personality disorders requires a nuanced approach that includes both pharmacotherapy and psychotherapy, as well as interdisciplinary care models.

This chapter will cover the **understanding of personality disorders and their diagnostic criteria**, explore the role of **pharmacotherapy and psychotherapy**, and highlight the importance of **collaborative care models**, including the role of **pharmacist practitioners** in supporting individuals with personality disorders.

12.1. Understanding Personality Disorders and Diagnostic Criteria

Personality disorders represent deeply ingrained, enduring patterns of behavior, cognition, and inner experience that deviate markedly from the expectations of an individual's culture. These patterns are rigid, pervasive, and lead to distress or impairment in various aspects of functioning.

According to the **DSM-5**, personality disorders are categorized into **three clusters**, each defined by a common theme of behaviors, thoughts, and emotions. These clusters help organize personality disorders based on their characteristic features and similarities.

12.1.1. Cluster A: Odd or Eccentric Disorders

Cluster A personality disorders are characterized by **odd**, **eccentric**, or **unusual thinking** and behavior patterns. Individuals with these disorders often exhibit **social detachment** and have difficulties in forming close relationships. Their thoughts and behaviors tend to be suspicious, detached, or distorted.

Paranoid Personality Disorder (PPD)

Paranoid Personality Disorder involves pervasive **distrust** and **suspicion** of others, where individuals believe, without sufficient basis, that others are trying to deceive, harm, or exploit them.

DSM-5 Diagnostic Criteria:

- **A.** A pervasive distrust and suspiciousness of others such that their motives are interpreted as malevolent, beginning by early adulthood and present in a variety of contexts, as indicated by **four (or more)** of the following:

- Suspects, without sufficient basis, that others are exploiting, harming, or deceiving them.
- Preoccupied with unjustified doubts about the loyalty or trustworthiness of friends or associates.
- Reluctant to confide in others because of an unwarranted fear that the information will be used maliciously against them.
- Reads hidden demeaning or threatening meanings into benign remarks or events.
- Persistently bears grudges (e.g., unforgiving of insults or slights).
- Perceives attacks on their character or reputation that are not apparent to others and is quick to react angrily or counterattack.
- Has recurrent suspicions, without justification, regarding the fidelity of their spouse or sexual partner.

Schizoid Personality Disorder (SPD)

Schizoid Personality Disorder is marked by **detachment from social relationships** and a **restricted range of emotional expression**. Individuals with this disorder tend to avoid social interaction, prefer solitude, and appear emotionally cold or indifferent.

DSM-5 Diagnostic Criteria:

- **A.** A pervasive pattern of detachment from social relationships and a restricted range of expression of emotions in interpersonal settings, beginning by early adulthood and present in a variety of contexts, as indicated by **four (or more)** of the following:
    - Neither desires nor enjoys close relationships, including being part of a family.
    - Almost always chooses solitary activities.
    - Has little, if any, interest in having sexual experiences with another person.
    - Takes pleasure in few, if any, activities.
    - Lacks close friends or confidants other than first-degree relatives.
    - Appears indifferent to praise or criticism from others.
    - Shows emotional coldness, detachment, or flattened affectivity.

Schizotypal Personality Disorder (STPD)

Schizotypal Personality Disorder is characterized by **eccentric behaviors**, **cognitive or perceptual distortions**, and marked social and interpersonal deficits. These individuals may engage in **magical thinking**, have **odd beliefs**, or exhibit **peculiar speech**.

DSM-5 Diagnostic Criteria:

- **A.** A pervasive pattern of social and interpersonal deficits marked by acute discomfort with, and reduced capacity for, close relationships, as well as by cognitive or perceptual distortions and eccentricities of behavior, beginning by early adulthood and present in a variety of contexts, as indicated by **five (or more)** of the following:
    - Ideas of reference (excluding delusions of reference).

- Odd beliefs or magical thinking that influences behavior (e.g., superstitions, telepathy).
- Unusual perceptual experiences, including bodily illusions.
- Odd thinking and speech (e.g., vague, metaphorical).
- Suspiciousness or paranoid ideation.
- Inappropriate or constricted affect.
- Behavior or appearance that is odd, eccentric, or peculiar.
- Lack of close friends or confidants other than first-degree relatives.
- Excessive social anxiety that does not diminish with familiarity.

12.2.2. Cluster B: Dramatic, Emotional, or Erratic Disorders

Cluster B personality disorders are marked by **dramatic, emotional,** or **unpredictable behaviors**. Individuals with these disorders may struggle with **impulse control, emotional regulation**, and maintaining stable relationships.

Borderline Personality Disorder (BPD)

Borderline Personality Disorder is characterized by **instability** in interpersonal relationships, self-image, and affect, along with marked **impulsivity**. Individuals may have an intense fear of abandonment, **emotional instability**, and engage in **self-harming behaviors**.

DSM-5 Diagnostic Criteria:

- **A.** A pervasive pattern of instability of interpersonal relationships, self-image, and affects, and marked impulsivity, beginning by early adulthood and present in a variety of contexts, as indicated by **five (or more)** of the following:
    - Frantic efforts to avoid real or imagined abandonment.
    - A pattern of unstable and intense interpersonal relationships characterized by alternating between extremes of idealization and devaluation.
    - Identity disturbance: markedly and persistently unstable self-image or sense of self.
    - Impulsivity in at least two areas that are potentially self-damaging (e.g., spending, sex, substance abuse, reckless driving, binge eating).
    - Recurrent suicidal behavior, gestures, or threats, or self-mutilating behavior.
    - Affective instability due to a marked reactivity of mood (e.g., intense episodic dysphoria, irritability, or anxiety).
    - Chronic feelings of emptiness.
    - Inappropriate, intense anger or difficulty controlling anger.
    - Transient, stress-related paranoid ideation or severe dissociative symptoms.

Antisocial Personality Disorder (ASPD)

Antisocial Personality Disorder involves a pervasive pattern of **disregard for the rights of others**, often violating social norms and engaging in **manipulative** or **reckless behaviors**.

DSM-5 Diagnostic Criteria:

- **A.** A pervasive pattern of disregard for and violation of the rights of others, occurring since age **15 years**, as indicated by **three (or more)** of the following:
    - Failure to conform to social norms with respect to lawful behaviors, repeatedly performing acts that are grounds for arrest.
    - Deceitfulness, as indicated by repeated lying, use of aliases, or conning others for personal profit or pleasure.
    - Impulsivity or failure to plan ahead.
    - Irritability and aggressiveness, as indicated by repeated physical fights or assaults.
    - Reckless disregard for the safety of self or others.
    - Consistent irresponsibility, as indicated by repeated failure to sustain consistent work behavior or honor financial obligations.
    - Lack of remorse, as indicated by being indifferent to or rationalizing having hurt, mistreated, or stolen from another.
- **B.** The individual is at least **18 years** of age.
- **C.** There is evidence of **conduct disorder** with onset before age 15.

Histrionic Personality Disorder (HPD)

Histrionic Personality Disorder involves excessive **emotional expression** and **attention-seeking behaviors**. Individuals with this disorder often display **dramatic** behaviors to gain approval and validation from others.

DSM-5 Diagnostic Criteria:

- **A.** A pervasive pattern of excessive emotionality and attention-seeking, beginning by early adulthood and present in a variety of contexts, as indicated by **five (or more)** of the following:
    - Is uncomfortable in situations in which they are not the center of attention.
    - Interaction with others is often characterized by inappropriate sexually seductive or provocative behavior.
    - Displays rapidly shifting and shallow expression of emotions.
    - Consistently uses physical appearance to draw attention to self.
    - Has a style of speech that is excessively impressionistic and lacking in detail.
    - Shows self-dramatization, theatricality, and exaggerated expression of emotion.
    - Is suggestible (i.e., easily influenced by others or circumstances).
    - Considers relationships to be more intimate than they actually are.

Narcissistic Personality Disorder (NPD)

Narcissistic Personality Disorder is marked by **grandiosity**, a need for **admiration**, and a lack of **empathy** for others. Individuals often have an inflated sense of self-importance and may exploit others for personal gain.

DSM-5 Diagnostic Criteria:

- **A.** A pervasive pattern of grandiosity (in fantasy or behavior), need for admiration, and lack of empathy, beginning by early adulthood and present in a variety of contexts, as indicated by **five (or more)** of the following:
    - Has a grandiose sense of self-importance (e.g., exaggerates achievements and talents, expects to be recognized as superior without commensurate achievements).
    - Is preoccupied with fantasies of unlimited success, power, brilliance, beauty, or ideal love.
    - Believes that they are "special" and unique and can only be understood by, or should associate with, other special or high-status people (or institutions).
    - Requires excessive admiration.
    - Has a sense of entitlement (i.e., unreasonable expectations of especially favorable treatment or automatic compliance with their expectations).
    - Is interpersonally exploitative (i.e., takes advantage of others to achieve their own ends).
    - Lacks empathy: is unwilling to recognize or identify with the feelings and needs of others.
    - Is often envious of others or believes that others are envious of them.
    - Shows arrogant, haughty behaviors or attitudes.

12.1.3. Cluster C: Anxious or Fearful Disorders

Cluster C personality disorders are characterized by **anxiety**, **fearfulness**, and behaviors aimed at avoiding **criticism**, **rejection**, or **separation**.

Avoidant Personality Disorder (AvPD)

Avoidant Personality Disorder involves extreme **social inhibition**, feelings of **inadequacy**, and **hypersensitivity to criticism** or rejection. Individuals often avoid social situations due to fear of being embarrassed or disliked.

DSM-5 Diagnostic Criteria:

- **A.** A pervasive pattern of social inhibition, feelings of inadequacy, and hypersensitivity to negative evaluation, beginning by early adulthood and present in a variety of contexts, as indicated by **four (or more)** of the following:
    - Avoids occupational activities that involve significant interpersonal contact because of fears of criticism, disapproval, or rejection.
    - Is unwilling to get involved with people unless certain of being liked.
    - Shows restraint within intimate relationships because of the fear of being shamed or ridiculed.

- Is preoccupied with being criticized or rejected in social situations.
- Is inhibited in new interpersonal situations because of feelings of inadequacy.
- Views self as socially inept, personally unappealing, or inferior to others.
- Is unusually reluctant to take personal risks or to engage in any new activities because they may prove embarrassing.

Dependent Personality Disorder (DPD)

Dependent Personality Disorder is marked by an excessive need to be **taken care of**, leading to **submissive**, **clingy** behavior and **fear of separation**. Individuals with DPD have difficulty making decisions independently and often defer to others.

DSM-5 Diagnostic Criteria:

- **A.** A pervasive and excessive need to be taken care of that leads to submissive and clinging behavior and fears of separation, beginning by early adulthood and present in a variety of contexts, as indicated by **five (or more)** of the following:
  - Has difficulty making everyday decisions without an excessive amount of advice and reassurance from others.
  - Needs others to assume responsibility for most major areas of their life.
  - Has difficulty expressing disagreement with others because of fear of loss of support or approval.
  - Has difficulty initiating projects or doing things on their own (because of a lack of self-confidence in judgment or abilities rather than a lack of motivation or energy).
  - Goes to excessive lengths to obtain nurturance and support from others, to the point of volunteering to do things that are unpleasant.
  - Feels uncomfortable or helpless when alone because of exaggerated fears of being unable to care for themselves.
  - Urgently seeks another relationship as a source of care and support when a close relationship ends.
  - Is unrealistically preoccupied with fears of being left to take care of themselves.

Obsessive-Compulsive Personality Disorder (OCPD)

Obsessive-Compulsive Personality Disorder is characterized by a preoccupation with **orderliness**, **perfectionism**, and control at the expense of flexibility, openness, and efficiency. Individuals with OCPD are overly focused on rules and details.

DSM-5 Diagnostic Criteria:

- **A.** A pervasive pattern of preoccupation with orderliness, perfectionism, and mental and interpersonal control, at the expense of flexibility, openness, and efficiency, beginning by early adulthood and present in a variety of contexts, as indicated by **four (or more)** of the following:

- Is preoccupied with details, rules, lists, order, organization, or schedules to the extent that the major point of the activity is lost.
- Shows perfectionism that interferes with task completion (e.g., is unable to complete a project because their own overly strict standards are not met).
- Is excessively devoted to work and productivity to the exclusion of leisure activities and friendships (not accounted for by obvious economic necessity).
- Is overconscientious, scrupulous, and inflexible about matters of morality, ethics, or values (not accounted for by cultural or religious identification).
- Is unable to discard worn-out or worthless objects even when they have no sentimental value.
- Is reluctant to delegate tasks or to work with others unless they submit to exactly their way of doing things.
- Adopts a miserly spending style toward both self and others; money is viewed as something to be hoarded for future catastrophes.
- Shows rigidity and stubbornness.

12.2. Treatment: Pharmacotherapy and Psychotherapy in Managing Personality Disorders

Treating **personality disorders** can be particularly challenging because these disorders involve deeply ingrained patterns of thinking, feeling, and behaving, which are often resistant to change. **Psychotherapy** is the primary treatment modality for most personality disorders, focusing on altering maladaptive behaviors and improving interpersonal functioning.

However, **pharmacotherapy** can also play a significant role in managing specific symptoms such as **mood instability**, **impulsivity**, and **anxiety**, or in addressing **comorbid conditions** like depression or anxiety disorders.

12.2.1. Pharmacotherapy for Personality Disorders

Pharmacotherapy in the treatment of personality disorders is **symptom-targeted** rather than aimed at curing the disorder itself. Medications are used to manage **specific symptoms** that interfere with functioning or contribute to emotional dysregulation, such as **impulsivity**, **anxiety**, or **depression**. Below are the primary pharmacological agents used to treat these symptoms in individuals with personality disorders.

Antidepressants

Selective Serotonin Reuptake Inhibitors (SSRIs) are commonly used to manage **mood symptoms**, including **depression**, **anxiety**, and **impulsivity**, in individuals with personality disorders. By increasing the availability of **serotonin** in the brain, SSRIs can stabilize mood and reduce the frequency of impulsive behaviors.

- **Targeted Symptoms**:
  - Depression, anxiety, emotional dysregulation, and impulsivity.

- **Common Uses**:
  - **Borderline Personality Disorder (BPD)**: SSRIs like **fluoxetine** and **sertraline** are frequently used to reduce **mood swings, anxiety,** and **impulsive behaviors** in individuals with BPD. While not specifically targeting the core features of the disorder, SSRIs can help stabilize emotions and improve daily functioning.
  - **Avoidant Personality Disorder (AvPD)**: In avoidant personality disorder, SSRIs may be used to manage **social anxiety** and **hypersensitivity to rejection**.
- **Examples**:
  - **Fluoxetine (Prozac)**: Often used to manage mood instability and impulsivity.
  - **Sertraline (Zoloft)**: Commonly used for its effects on both depression and anxiety.
- **Clinical Considerations**:
  - SSRIs are generally **well-tolerated** and can be useful in individuals with **comorbid depression** or **anxiety disorders**. However, they may take several weeks to take full effect and can cause side effects such as **sexual dysfunction, nausea,** and **insomnia**.

Mood Stabilizers

Mood stabilizers, such as **lithium** and certain **anticonvulsants** (e.g., **valproate, lamotrigine**), are used to help manage **mood swings** and **impulsivity**, particularly in individuals with **borderline personality disorder** or **antisocial personality disorder**.

- **Targeted Symptoms**:
  - **Emotional dysregulation, mood swings,** and **impulsive behaviors**.
- **Common Uses**:
  - **Borderline Personality Disorder (BPD)**: Mood stabilizers like **lamotrigine** can help reduce **mood lability** and **impulsivity**, improving emotional stability.
  - **Antisocial Personality Disorder (ASPD)**: Mood stabilizers may also be used to manage **aggression** and **impulsivity** in individuals with ASPD, though the evidence is less clear.
- **Examples**:
  - **Lithium**: Often used to manage mood instability and reduce aggressive or impulsive behavior.
  - **Valproate (Depakote)** and **lamotrigine (Lamictal)**: Anticonvulsants that can be helpful in stabilizing mood and reducing impulsivity.
- **Clinical Considerations**:
  - These medications require careful monitoring, particularly **lithium**, which has a narrow therapeutic window and can cause **toxicity**. **Valproate** and **lamotrigine** are typically well-tolerated but may carry risks of **rash** or **liver toxicity**.

Antipsychotics

Atypical antipsychotics are often used in **low doses** to address **psychotic-like symptoms** (e.g., paranoia, severe mood dysregulation) in individuals with personality disorders, particularly in **schizotypal** or **borderline personality disorder**. These medications can also be helpful in managing **emotional instability** and **impulsive behaviors**.

- **Targeted Symptoms**:
  - **Paranoia**, **psychotic-like symptoms**, **severe mood dysregulation**, and **impulsivity**.
- **Common Uses**:
  - **Schizotypal Personality Disorder (STPD)**: Low-dose **atypical antipsychotics** like **aripiprazole** or **quetiapine** may be used to reduce **paranoia** and **magical thinking**, common in schizotypal personality disorder.
  - **Borderline Personality Disorder (BPD)**: Atypical antipsychotics may help manage **severe emotional dysregulation** and reduce **impulsivity**.
- **Examples**:
  - **Aripiprazole (Abilify)**: Often used for its mood-stabilizing and antipsychotic properties.
  - **Quetiapine (Seroquel)**: Commonly used in lower doses to manage mood swings and reduce impulsive behavior.
- **Clinical Considerations**:
  - **Atypical antipsychotics** are associated with side effects such as **weight gain**, **metabolic syndrome**, and **sedation**. Careful monitoring of metabolic health (e.g., blood glucose, lipid levels) is recommended, especially with long-term use.)

Anxiolytics

Benzodiazepines may be used cautiously for the short-term management of **severe anxiety** in individuals with **Cluster C personality disorders** (e.g., **avoidant personality disorder**, **dependent personality disorder**). However, these medications carry a risk of **dependence** and should be avoided in individuals with **impulsivity** or a history of **substance use**.

- **Targeted Symptoms**:
  - **Acute anxiety**, **panic**, and **social anxiety**.
- **Common Uses**:
  - **Avoidant Personality Disorder (AvPD)**: Benzodiazepines like **lorazepam** may be used short-term to manage **social anxiety** or **acute distress**.
  - **Dependent Personality Disorder (DPD)**: In rare cases, benzodiazepines may be used to manage **anxiety** in individuals with DPD, but caution is advised due to the potential for **dependency**.
- **Examples**:
  - **Lorazepam (Ativan)**: A short-acting benzodiazepine used to manage acute anxiety.
  - **Clonazepam (Klonopin)**: A longer-acting option for anxiety management.
- **Clinical Considerations**:
  - Benzodiazepines should be used **sparingly** and for **short durations** due to the risk of **tolerance**, **dependence**, and **withdrawal symptoms**. They are generally

avoided in personality disorders characterized by **impulsivity** or a history of **substance abuse**.

12.2.2. Psychotherapy for Personality Disorders

Psychotherapy remains the cornerstone of treatment for **personality disorders**, as it directly targets the maladaptive behaviors, thought patterns, and interpersonal difficulties that characterize these conditions. Several evidence-based psychotherapies have been developed to help individuals with personality disorders build healthier coping strategies and improve emotional regulation, interpersonal relationships, and overall functioning.

Dialectical Behavior Therapy (DBT)

Dialectical Behavior Therapy (DBT) was originally developed for **borderline personality disorder (BPD)** and has since become one of the most effective treatments for this condition. DBT combines elements of **cognitive-behavioral therapy (CBT)** with mindfulness techniques to help individuals manage intense emotions and impulsive behaviors.

- **Core Components**:
    - **Emotion Regulation**: Teaching individuals how to manage and reduce emotional intensity.
    - **Distress Tolerance**: Helping patients develop skills to tolerate and survive crises without resorting to self-harm or other maladaptive behaviors.
    - **Interpersonal Effectiveness**: Teaching communication and relationship skills to improve social interactions.
    - **Mindfulness**: Helping individuals focus on the present moment and observe their emotions and thoughts without judgment.
- **Effectiveness**:
    - **DBT** has been shown to significantly reduce **self-harming behaviors**, improve **mood regulation**, and reduce the frequency of **hospitalizations** in individuals with BPD. It is also effective in treating **suicidal ideation**.

Cognitive-Behavioral Therapy (CBT)

Cognitive-Behavioral Therapy (CBT) helps individuals identify and challenge **distorted thinking patterns** and develop **healthier coping strategies**. CBT is commonly used for **avoidant**, **obsessive-compulsive**, and **paranoid personality disorders**.

- **Core Components**:
    - **Cognitive Restructuring**: Identifying and changing negative thought patterns.
    - **Behavioral Activation**: Encouraging individuals to engage in positive, goal-oriented behaviors.
    - **Exposure Therapy**: Gradual exposure to feared situations to reduce avoidance.
- **Effectiveness**:

- CBT has been shown to reduce **social anxiety** and improve **self-esteem** in individuals with **avoidant personality disorder**. It is also effective in treating **obsessive-compulsive behaviors** in **obsessive-compulsive personality disorder (OCPD)**.

Mentalization-Based Therapy (MBT)

Mentalization-Based Therapy (MBT) is designed to help individuals with **borderline personality disorder (BPD)** develop the ability to **mentalize**, or understand their own and others' thoughts and feelings. This improves **emotional regulation** and helps individuals build more stable interpersonal relationships.

- **Core Components**:
    - **Mentalizing**: Developing insight into one's thoughts and emotions, as well as understanding others' perspectives.
    - **Interpersonal Focus**: Improving relationships by recognizing and correcting misinterpretations of others' intentions.
- **Effectiveness**:
    - **MBT** has been shown to improve **emotional regulation** and reduce **self-harming behaviors** in individuals with BPD. It also helps improve **interpersonal relationships** and reduces emotional reactivity.

Schema-Focused Therapy

Schema-Focused Therapy (SFT) addresses **early maladaptive schemas**, which are deeply held negative beliefs about oneself and the world that are often formed during childhood. These schemas contribute to problematic behaviors and emotions in personality disorders.

- **Core Components**:
    - **Identifying Maladaptive Schemas**: Recognizing deeply rooted negative beliefs (e.g., "I am unlovable").
    - **Reframing Schemas**: Challenging and modifying maladaptive schemas through cognitive restructuring.
    - **Behavioral Change**: Encouraging individuals to develop healthier ways of interacting with others and coping with emotional distress.
- **Effectiveness**:
    - **SFT** has been particularly useful for individuals with **narcissistic, borderline,** and **avoidant personality disorders**, helping them change deeply ingrained beliefs and improve overall functioning.

12.3. Collaborative Care Models and Role of Pharmacist Practitioners in Supporting Individuals with Personality Disorders

12.3.1. Collaborative Care Models:

Personality disorders often require a **multidisciplinary approach**, involving psychiatrists, psychologists, social workers, nurses, and **pharmacists**. Collaborative care models are essential in addressing the **complex needs** of individuals with personality disorders, as they often require integrated medical, psychological, and social support.

- **Psychiatrists and Primary Care Providers**: Psychiatrists oversee pharmacological treatment, manage co-occurring mental health disorders, and work alongside primary care providers to address physical health needs. For example, individuals with **antisocial personality disorder** may present with substance use disorders, requiring coordinated care between addiction specialists and mental health professionals.
- **Psychologists and Therapists**: Psychologists provide **psychotherapy** and conduct psychological assessments to identify the most appropriate therapeutic interventions for each individual. Long-term psychotherapy, such as **DBT** or **schema-focused therapy**, may be conducted in individual or group settings.
- **Social Workers**: Social workers help connect individuals with social services, housing, and vocational training. They often play a critical role in addressing the **social determinants of health**, which can exacerbate personality disorder symptoms, such as housing instability or unemployment.

12.3.2. Role of Advanced Pharmacist Practitioners:

Pharmacists and **advanced pharmacist practitioners** are key members of the collaborative care team, particularly in **medication management**, patient education, and monitoring for side effects.

- **Medication Management**: Pharmacists help optimize medication regimens for individuals with personality disorders by ensuring appropriate dosing, addressing potential drug interactions, and recommending adjustments based on efficacy and side effects. For example, pharmacists can help manage **polypharmacy** in individuals with comorbid mood disorders, anxiety, or substance use disorders.
- **Patient Education**: Pharmacist practitioners provide education about the **importance of medication adherence**, the **side effects** of psychotropic medications, and strategies to minimize those side effects. Individuals with personality disorders may struggle with **impulsivity**, making adherence to long-term pharmacotherapy challenging.
- **Monitoring for Adverse Effects**: Pharmacists play a role in monitoring patients for adverse effects, such as **weight gain**, **metabolic changes**, or **cardiovascular risks** associated with antipsychotic medications. They can also help mitigate the side effects of **mood stabilizers** and **antidepressants**, improving overall patient outcomes.

Personality disorders are complex and deeply ingrained psychiatric conditions that significantly impact interpersonal functioning and quality of life. Managing these disorders requires a comprehensive treatment approach that includes **psychotherapy**, **pharmacotherapy**, and **collaborative care**.

Psychotherapies such as **DBT** and **CBT** are critical for addressing the cognitive and emotional patterns underlying these disorders, while medications can help manage specific symptoms such as mood instability and impulsivity.

Collaborative care models that integrate the expertise of psychiatrists, psychologists, pharmacists, and social workers provide the best support for individuals with personality disorders. Pharmacist practitioners, in particular, play a vital role in optimizing medication regimens, educating patients, and ensuring long-term adherence to treatment plans.

12.4. ICD-10 for Personality Disorders

These ICD-10 codes cover a range of personality disorders categorized into clusters A, B, and C, and are used for diagnosis and treatment planning in clinical settings.

Cluster A: Odd or Eccentric Disorders

1. **F60.0** – Paranoid Personality Disorder
2. **F60.1** – Schizoid Personality Disorder
3. **F21** – Schizotypal Disorder (Schizotypal Personality Disorder is included here in ICD-10)

Cluster B: Dramatic, Emotional, or Erratic Disorders

1. **F60.2** – Antisocial Personality Disorder
2. **F60.3** – Borderline Personality Disorder
3. **F60.4** – Histrionic Personality Disorder
4. **F60.81** – Narcissistic Personality Disorder

Cluster C: Anxious or Fearful Disorders

1. **F60.6** – Avoidant (Anxious) Personality Disorder
2. **F60.7** – Dependent Personality Disorder
3. **F60.5** – Obsessive-Compulsive Personality Disorder (OCPD)

Other Personality Disorders

1. **F60.89** – Other specific personality disorders
2. **F60.9** – Personality Disorder, unspecified

References:

1. American Psychiatric Association. (2013). *Diagnostic and Statistical Manual of Mental Disorders* (5th ed.).
2. Linehan, M. M., Schmidt, H., Dimeff, L. A., et al. (1999). Dialectical behavior therapy for patients with borderline personality disorder and drug-dependence. *American Journal on Addictions*, 8(4), 279-292.

3. Paris, J. (2015). Pharmacotherapy of personality disorders: Evidence and practice. *Current Psychiatry Reports*, 17(1), 550.
4. McMain, S. F., Links, P. S., Gnam, W. H., et al. (2009). A randomized trial of dialectical behavior therapy versus general psychiatric management for borderline personality disorder. *American Journal of Psychiatry*, 166(12), 1365-1374.
5. Bateman, A., & Fonagy, P. (2010). Mentalization based treatment for borderline personality disorder. *World Psychiatry*, 9(1), 11-15.
6. Sperry, L., & Sperry, J. A. (2016). **Handbook of Diagnosis and Treatment of DSM-5 Personality Disorders**. New York, NY: Routledge.
7. Zanarini, M. C., Frankenburg, F. R., Reich, D. B., et al. (2005). Treatment of borderline personality disorder with olanzapine: A double-blind, placebo-controlled pilot study. *American Journal of Psychiatry*, 160(4), 563-569.

Chapter 13: Geriatric Psychiatry

As the global population ages, the prevalence of psychiatric disorders in older adults is increasing, presenting unique challenges in diagnosis and treatment. Managing psychiatric disorders in this population requires special consideration due to age-related physiological changes, the presence of multiple comorbidities, and the increased risk of adverse effects from medications.

This chapter explores the **special considerations in managing psychiatric disorders in older adults**, addresses **pharmacotherapy challenges and considerations**, and provides **medication management strategies** to optimize safety and efficacy. It also discusses the importance of **addressing polypharmacy** and managing **drug interactions** in older adults with psychiatric conditions.

13.1. Special Considerations in Managing Psychiatric Disorders in Older Adults

Managing psychiatric disorders in older adults requires special attention to the unique biological, psychological, and social factors associated with aging. The interplay between physical health, cognitive decline, sensory impairments, and changes in social roles can complicate the assessment and treatment of psychiatric conditions in this population.

13.1.1. Aging and Mental Health

The aging process involves numerous changes that influence mental health. Older adults often experience **cognitive decline, sensory impairments, reduced mobility,** and **social role changes**. These factors can either precipitate or exacerbate psychiatric disorders such as **depression, anxiety,** and **dementia**.

Cognitive Changes

- **Cognitive decline** is a normal part of aging, but distinguishing between typical age-related changes and pathological conditions is critical. **Mild cognitive impairment (MCI)** is an intermediate stage between normal cognitive aging and **dementia**, and in some cases, it progresses to conditions such as **Alzheimer's disease** or **vascular dementia**.
- **Alzheimer's disease** and **vascular dementia** are common forms of dementia that profoundly affect an individual's mood, behavior, and overall functioning.
- Differentiating between cognitive impairment and psychiatric conditions like **late-onset depression** is essential for accurate diagnosis. In some cases, **depression** can manifest with cognitive symptoms, leading to **pseudodementia**, where cognitive decline is secondary to depressive symptoms.

Sensory Loss and Isolation

- **Hearing loss** and **vision impairments** are prevalent in older adults, contributing to **social isolation**, which can, in turn, exacerbate **depression** and **anxiety**. These sensory deficits can also complicate communication during psychiatric evaluations, making it difficult to accurately assess cognitive and emotional states.
- **Isolation** stemming from sensory loss can lead to a further decline in cognitive function and mental health, as social engagement is a protective factor against cognitive decline and mood disorders.

Comorbidities

- Older adults commonly have multiple chronic health conditions (e.g., **hypertension**, **diabetes**, **heart disease**), which complicate the management of psychiatric disorders. **Polypharmacy** (use of multiple medications) is common in older adults and increases the risk of adverse drug interactions that can affect both mental and physical health.
- Psychiatric symptoms, such as **fatigue** and **anhedonia** in depression, can overlap with symptoms of physical illnesses like **heart failure**, making diagnosis more challenging.

13.1.2. Depression and Anxiety in Older Adults

Late-Onset Depression

- **Depression** is one of the most common psychiatric disorders in older adults, with many individuals experiencing their first depressive episode later in life. **Late-onset depression** is often linked to **neurodegenerative processes**, **vascular changes**, and psychosocial stressors such as **bereavement**, **retirement**, or **chronic illness**.
- In older adults, depression may present with **cognitive symptoms**, such as **poor concentration**, **memory difficulties**, and **slowed thinking**. These symptoms may be mistaken for **dementia**, leading to the diagnosis of **pseudodementia**, where cognitive impairment is secondary to depressive symptoms.
- Older adults are also more likely to experience **somatic symptoms** of depression, such as **pain**, **fatigue**, or **appetite changes**, which may complicate the clinical picture.

Anxiety Disorders

- **Anxiety** is also common in older adults and frequently co-occurs with **depression**. The most common anxiety disorders in this population include **generalized anxiety disorder (GAD)** and **panic disorder**.
- Anxiety in older adults may manifest more with **physical symptoms**, such as **chest pain**, **shortness of breath**, or **gastrointestinal disturbances**, which can easily be mistaken for medical conditions like **cardiac** or **gastrointestinal disorders**.
- Older adults with anxiety disorders are at higher risk of developing **insomnia**, **social isolation**, and **functional impairment**, all of which can worsen both physical and mental health outcomes.

13.1.3. Psychotic Disorders and Delirium

Psychotic Disorders

- Psychotic symptoms may arise in older adults due to various causes, including **delirium**, **dementia**, or primary psychiatric conditions such as **schizophrenia** or **delusional disorder**.
- **Delirium** is an acute, fluctuating change in cognition and attention that is particularly common in hospitalized older adults. It can be triggered by factors such as **infections**, **medications**, or **metabolic imbalances** and requires immediate medical attention.
- **Delusional disorder** in older adults may manifest as **paranoia** or **persecutory delusions**, where the individual believes others are trying to harm them, often without sufficient evidence.

Dementia-Related Psychosis

- Individuals with **Alzheimer's disease** or **Lewy body dementia** often develop **psychotic symptoms**, including **paranoia**, **hallucinations**, and **delusions**. These symptoms can be particularly distressing for both the patient and caregivers and require careful management.
- Differentiating between **dementia-related psychosis** and psychosis due to primary psychiatric conditions is essential for proper treatment. In dementia-related psychosis, the focus is often on managing symptoms without exacerbating cognitive decline, which can occur with some antipsychotic medications.

Delirium

- **Delirium** is an acute confusional state with fluctuating levels of consciousness, attention, and cognition. It is commonly seen in hospitalized older adults, especially those with underlying cognitive impairment or sensory deficits.
- Delirium is often caused by **infections**, **medications**, **metabolic disturbances**, or surgery, and it is a medical emergency that requires prompt identification and treatment. Delirium can easily be mistaken for dementia or psychiatric disorders, so it is essential to carefully assess its onset, duration, and associated symptoms.

13.2. Treatment Challenges and Considerations in Geriatric Psychiatry

13.2.1. Age-Related Physiological Changes:

Pharmacokinetics and pharmacodynamics are altered in older adults due to changes in body composition, liver function, kidney function, and receptor sensitivity. These changes necessitate adjustments in medication dosing and selection to avoid adverse effects.

- **Absorption and Distribution**: Age-related decreases in **gastric motility** and **blood flow** can affect drug absorption, while increased **body fat** and decreased **lean body mass** alter the distribution of lipophilic drugs (e.g., benzodiazepines), leading to

prolonged effects. **Water-soluble medications** may have reduced volume of distribution, increasing their plasma concentration.
- **Metabolism and Excretion**: Reduced **hepatic metabolism** and **renal clearance** in older adults can lead to drug accumulation, particularly for medications metabolized by the **cytochrome P450** system or excreted via the kidneys (e.g., lithium, digoxin). Monitoring liver and kidney function is critical when prescribing psychotropic medications.

13.2.2. Increased Sensitivity to Medications:

Older adults are more sensitive to the effects of psychotropic medications, particularly **sedatives**, **antipsychotics**, and **anticholinergics**, increasing the risk of **falls**, **delirium**, **cognitive decline**, and **orthostatic hypotension**. Benzodiazepines and **anticholinergic agents** should be avoided or used with extreme caution due to their association with cognitive impairment and fall risk.

- **Benzodiazepines**: While effective for acute anxiety or insomnia, benzodiazepines are associated with increased risk of **sedation**, **confusion**, **falls**, and **dependence** in older adults. Alternatives such as **SSRIs** or **cognitive behavioral therapy for insomnia (CBT-I)** are preferred.
- **Antipsychotics**: **Atypical antipsychotics** (e.g., **quetiapine**, **risperidone**) are often used for treating psychosis or agitation in dementia, but they carry a **black box warning** due to increased mortality from cardiovascular and infectious causes in older adults with dementia.

13.3. Medication Management Strategies to Optimize Safety and Efficacy

Given the increased risks associated with pharmacotherapy in older adults, thoughtful strategies must be employed to ensure both the safety and efficacy of psychotropic medications. Age-related physiological changes, polypharmacy, and increased sensitivity to side effects make this population particularly vulnerable to adverse drug events. The following strategies are essential for optimizing medication management in geriatric psychiatry.

13.3.1. Start Low, Go Slow

The principle of "start low, go slow" is critical when prescribing psychotropic medications to older adults. This approach involves initiating treatment at **lower doses** than those typically prescribed to younger patients and **slowly titrating** the dose to reach therapeutic levels.

- **Rationale**:
    - **Pharmacokinetic changes** (e.g., decreased renal and hepatic function) and **pharmacodynamic changes** (e.g., increased receptor sensitivity) in older adults can lead to greater **drug accumulation** and **intensified effects**. Therefore, starting at a lower dose helps minimize the risk of **adverse drug reactions (ADRs)**.

- - **Gradual titration** allows clinicians to assess the **patient's response** to the medication while monitoring for potential side effects. Older adults may reach therapeutic benefits at doses lower than the standard recommended for younger populations.
- **Examples**:
  - **Antidepressants (SSRIs)**: Start with a lower dose (e.g., **sertraline 25 mg** instead of 50 mg) and increase gradually based on the patient's tolerance and clinical response.
  - **Antipsychotics (Atypical antipsychotics)**: For treating agitation in dementia, lower doses (e.g., **quetiapine 12.5–25 mg**) should be used initially, with careful monitoring for sedation, falls, and metabolic side effects.
- **Benefits**:
  - Reduces the risk of **sedation, falls, orthostatic hypotension**, and **cognitive impairment**, all of which are common adverse effects in older adults.
  - Improves patient **adherence** by minimizing the likelihood of intolerable side effects that might otherwise lead to discontinuation.

13.3.2. Regular Monitoring and Deprescribing

Regular **monitoring** is critical to ensure that medications prescribed to older adults remain effective and safe over time. Many older adults are prescribed psychotropic medications for prolonged periods, necessitating continuous assessment of **medication efficacy**, **side effects**, and **potential drug interactions**. For long-term use, **deprescribing** should be considered to reduce the risk of polypharmacy and adverse effects.

Monitoring Side Effects

- **Common Side Effects to Monitor**:
  - **Sedation**, which increases the risk of falls and fractures.
  - **Orthostatic hypotension**, leading to dizziness and syncope.
  - **Confusion** or **delirium**, which may mimic worsening dementia or cognitive decline.
  - **Weight gain** and **metabolic disturbances** (especially with antipsychotics).
- **Monitoring Specific Medications**:
  - **Lithium**: Regular monitoring of **serum lithium levels** is essential to avoid toxicity, especially in the presence of reduced renal clearance in older adults. **Thyroid** and **kidney function** should also be assessed periodically.
  - **Valproate**: Blood tests to monitor **valproate levels, liver function**, and **platelet count** are recommended to prevent hepatotoxicity and thrombocytopenia.

Deprescribing Guidelines

Deprescribing involves **tapering** or **discontinuing** medications that may no longer be necessary or may pose more risks than benefits. This process is particularly important for medications like **benzodiazepines**, **antipsychotics**, and **anticholinergics**, which are associated with **cognitive decline**, **falls**, and **dependence**.

- **Benzodiazepine Deprescribing**:
    - Benzodiazepines are commonly prescribed for **anxiety** or **insomnia** but carry significant risks in older adults, including **sedation**, **dependence**, **falls**, and **cognitive impairment**.
    - **Tapering** is the recommended approach to discontinuing benzodiazepines, as abrupt cessation can lead to **withdrawal symptoms** such as **anxiety**, **insomnia**, and **seizures**. A **slow taper** (e.g., 10–25% dose reduction every 1–2 weeks) allows the body to adjust gradually.
    - **Non-pharmacological interventions**, such as Cognitive Behavioral Therapy (**CBT**) for anxiety or **Cognitive Behavioral Therapy for Insomnia (CBT-I)**, can support benzodiazepine deprescribing by addressing the underlying conditions without the need for long-term medication use.
- **Antipsychotic Deprescribing**:
    - Antipsychotics are frequently used in older adults with **dementia-related psychosis** or **agitation**, but they increase the risk of **cardiovascular events**, **stroke**, and **mortality**.
    - **Tapering** should be gradual, and behavioral interventions should be implemented to manage agitation or psychosis in dementia.
- **Anticholinergic Deprescribing**:
    - **Anticholinergic medications** are linked to **cognitive decline**, **delirium**, and **urinary retention** in older adults. Gradually reducing these medications and replacing them with safer alternatives (if needed) is a critical strategy in geriatric care.

Deprescribing Considerations:

- **Patient-specific factors**, such as the presence of multiple comorbidities, cognitive function, and life expectancy, should guide the decision to deprescribe.
- **Communication** with the patient and caregivers is essential during the deprescribing process to set expectations, address concerns, and provide reassurance.

13.3.3. Individualized Treatment and Polypharmacy Management

In older adults, it is common to encounter **polypharmacy** (the use of five or more medications), which increases the risk of **adverse drug reactions**, **drug interactions**, and **medication non-adherence**. Therefore, it is essential to develop **individualized treatment plans** that minimize unnecessary medications while ensuring therapeutic goals are met.

Polypharmacy Management Strategies:

- **Comprehensive Medication Review**: Regularly review the patient's complete medication list, including **over-the-counter** and **herbal supplements**, to identify medications that may be contributing to side effects or are no longer necessary.
- **Medication Reconciliation**: Ensure that medications are accurately documented and reviewed during every clinical encounter, particularly after transitions of care (e.g., hospital discharge).
- **Prioritizing Non-Pharmacological Interventions**: In many cases, behavioral therapies and **lifestyle interventions** can be as effective as medications, particularly for conditions like **anxiety**, **insomnia**, and **mild depression**.

13.4. Non-Pharmacological Interventions and Psychotherapy

While medications play an important role in managing psychiatric conditions, **non-pharmacological approaches** are often equally effective and come without the side effects associated with psychotropic drugs. Behavioral therapies, especially **Cognitive Behavioral Therapy (CBT)**, can be particularly beneficial in older adults.

Cognitive Behavioral Therapy (CBT):

- **CBT for Anxiety and Depression**: In older adults, **CBT** can be effective in addressing **negative thought patterns**, **rumination**, and **avoidance behaviors**. It is especially valuable for managing **late-life depression** and **anxiety**, often providing a safer alternative to medication.
- **CBT for Insomnia (CBT-I)**: CBT-I is an evidence-based, non-pharmacological treatment for insomnia that has shown to be as effective as sleep medications in improving sleep quality. It focuses on modifying maladaptive sleep habits and addressing underlying causes of insomnia.

13.5. Caregiver Involvement and Education

In many cases, older adults may require **assistance with medication management**, either due to cognitive decline, physical limitations, or complex medication regimens. Involving **caregivers** and educating both the patient and caregivers about the importance of **adherence**, **monitoring** for side effects, and **non-pharmacological alternatives** is critical for optimizing medication safety.

Caregiver Education:

- Teach caregivers to recognize signs of **adverse drug reactions**, such as **confusion**, **falls**, or **worsening cognition**.
- Provide clear instructions on **medication administration** and **monitoring**, particularly for medications with a **narrow therapeutic index** (e.g., lithium).

13.6. Addressing Polypharmacy and Drug Interactions in Older Adults with Psychiatric Disorders

13.6.1. Polypharmacy:

Polypharmacy, defined as the use of five or more medications, is common in older adults due to the presence of multiple comorbidities. Polypharmacy increases the risk of **drug-drug interactions**, **adverse effects**, and **nonadherence**. Older adults with psychiatric disorders are particularly vulnerable to polypharmacy due to the frequent use of **psychotropic medications** alongside medications for physical health conditions (e.g., antihypertensives, antidiabetics).

- **Beers Criteria**: The **Beers Criteria**, published by the **American Geriatrics Society**, provides a list of medications that are potentially inappropriate for use in older adults due to their risk of adverse effects. Psychotropic medications, including **benzodiazepines**, **anticholinergics**, and **antipsychotics**, are prominently featured in these guidelines due to their potential for causing **cognitive impairment**, **falls**, and **delirium**.

13.6.2. Managing Drug Interactions:

Older adults are at higher risk for drug interactions due to the reduced capacity of the liver and kidneys to metabolize and excrete medications, as well as the frequent use of multiple medications.

- **Cytochrome P450 Interactions**: Many psychotropic medications are metabolized via the **CYP450 enzyme system**, which is also responsible for metabolizing a wide range of cardiovascular, gastrointestinal, and pain medications. **SSRIs**, **antipsychotics**, and **anticonvulsants** (e.g., **carbamazepine**) are particularly prone to interactions via CYP450 pathways. Monitoring for drug interactions and adjusting dosages when necessary is essential to avoid toxicity or reduced efficacy.
- **QT Prolongation**: Some psychotropic medications, such as **antipsychotics** (e.g., **quetiapine**, **haloperidol**) and certain **antidepressants** (e.g., **citalopram**), can prolong the **QT interval**, increasing the risk of **torsades de pointes** and other arrhythmias. ECG monitoring is advised, particularly in older adults with pre-existing cardiovascular conditions.

Managing psychiatric disorders in older adults requires special consideration due to age-related physiological changes, the risk of polypharmacy, and the presence of comorbidities. Pharmacotherapy should be approached cautiously, with close attention to dosing, side effects, and drug interactions.

Non-pharmacological interventions such as psychotherapy and lifestyle modifications play a key role in reducing the need for psychotropic medications and improving quality of life. **Collaborative care** involving psychiatrists, primary care providers, and pharmacists is essential for ensuring comprehensive, safe, and effective management of psychiatric conditions in the elderly.

References:

1. American Psychiatric Association. (2013). *Diagnostic and Statistical Manual of Mental Disorders* (5th ed.).
2. American Geriatrics Society. (2019). Updated AGS Beers Criteria for potentially inappropriate medication use in older adults. *Journal of the American Geriatrics Society*, 67(4), 674-694.
3. Maust, D. T., Kim, H. M., Seyfried, L. S., et al. (2015). Antipsychotics, other psychotropics, and the risk of death in patients with dementia: Number needed to harm. *JAMA Psychiatry*, 72(5), 438-445.
4. Wetherell, J. L., Lenze, E. J., Stanley, M. A., et al. (2005). Cognitive-behavioral therapy for generalized anxiety disorder in older adults: A randomized controlled trial. *JAMA*, 293(19), 2337-2346.
5. Hilmer, S. N., Gnjidic, D., & Le Couteur, D. G. (2012). Thinking through the medication list: Appropriate prescribing and deprescribing in robust and frail older patients. *Australian Family Physician*, 41(12), 924-928.
6. Lenze, E. J., & Wetherell, J. L. (2011). A lifespan view of anxiety disorders. *Dialogues in Clinical Neuroscience*, 13(4), 381-399.
7. Flint, A. J., & Gagnon, N. (2002). Diagnosis and management of generalized anxiety disorder in older adults. *CNS Drugs*, 16(6), 445-458.

Chapter 14: Pediatric Psychiatry

Pediatric psychiatry involves the diagnosis, treatment, and management of psychiatric disorders in children and adolescents. Early identification and intervention are critical in mitigating the long-term impact of these disorders, which can affect academic performance, social relationships, and emotional development.

This chapter provides an overview of **common psychiatric disorders in children and adolescents**, explores **pharmacotherapy considerations** and **evidence-based treatments**, addresses **monitoring for adverse effects** and optimizing medication regimens, and discusses the **role of pharmacist practitioners** in pediatric mental health care.

14.1. Common Psychiatric Disorders in Children and Adolescents

Children and adolescents often experience mental health challenges that require early identification and intervention.

The most common psychiatric disorders in this population include **Attention-Deficit/Hyperactivity Disorder (ADHD), anxiety disorders, depressive disorders, Autism Spectrum Disorder (ASD), Oppositional Defiant Disorder (ODD),** and **Conduct Disorder**. Each disorder presents with distinct features, diagnostic criteria, and potential comorbidities that must be considered in assessment and treatment.

14.1.1. Attention-Deficit/Hyperactivity Disorder (ADHD)

ADHD is one of the most common **neurodevelopmental disorders** in children, affecting their ability to focus, control impulses, and manage activity levels in an age-appropriate manner. It often leads to difficulties in academic, social, and family settings.

DSM-5 Diagnostic Criteria:

- The diagnosis of **ADHD** requires at least **six or more symptoms** of **inattention** and/or **hyperactivity-impulsivity** that persist for at least **six months** and are **inconsistent** with the child's developmental level.
- Symptoms must occur in **more than one setting** (e.g., home, school) and cause **significant impairment** in functioning.

Presentation Types:

1. **Predominantly Inattentive Type**:
    - Difficulty **sustaining attention**.
    - **Disorganization, forgetfulness**, and being easily distracted.
2. **Predominantly Hyperactive-Impulsive Type**:

- **Fidgeting**, **excessive talking**, and difficulty staying seated.
- **Impulsivity**: Acting without thinking, interrupting others, or difficulty waiting for turns.
3. **Combined Type**:
    - Symptoms of both **inattention** and **hyperactivity-impulsivity** are present.

Comorbidities:

- **ADHD** frequently co-occurs with other disorders, including:
    - **Learning disorders**
    - **Oppositional Defiant Disorder (ODD)**
    - **Anxiety disorders**

Impact:

ADHD can impair **academic performance**, **social relationships**, and family dynamics, often requiring a **multidisciplinary approach** that includes **behavioral therapy** and, in some cases, **medication management**.

14.1.2. Anxiety Disorders

Anxiety disorders in children and adolescents involve excessive worry, fear, or avoidance behaviors that interfere with **daily functioning**. These disorders often manifest as fears related to specific situations or concerns about separation from caregivers.

Common Anxiety Disorders:

- **Generalized Anxiety Disorder (GAD)**: Excessive worry about a variety of topics (e.g., school, health) that is difficult to control and leads to physical symptoms such as restlessness, fatigue, and irritability.
- **Separation Anxiety Disorder**:
    - **Excessive fear** or **anxiety** about separation from caregivers or home.
    - Most common in **younger children**, but can persist into adolescence.
    - May lead to **school refusal**, **clinginess**, or **nightmares** about separation.
- **Social Anxiety Disorder**:
    - Intense **fear of social situations** or **performance-based situations**, leading to avoidance of interactions where the child fears being **scrutinized** or **judged** by others.
    - Symptoms may include **blushing**, **sweating**, and **trembling** in social settings.

Impact:

Children with anxiety disorders often experience **academic difficulties**, avoidance of **social activities**, and problems with **peer relationships**. Early identification and **cognitive-behavioral therapy (CBT)** are effective treatments, and in some cases, **medication** may be needed.

14.1.3. Depressive Disorders

Depression in children and adolescents can present differently from adults, often with **irritability** and **withdrawal** rather than overt sadness. Early detection and intervention are crucial to prevent long-term consequences on emotional development.

Major Depressive Disorder (MDD):

- Persistent **low mood** or **irritability**, **loss of interest** in activities, changes in **appetite or sleep**, and feelings of **worthlessness** or **guilt**.
- Symptoms must persist for at least **two weeks**.
- In children, depression may manifest as **behavioral problems**, declining **academic performance**, or **social withdrawal** rather than sadness.

Disruptive Mood Dysregulation Disorder (DMDD):

- DMDD is characterized by **chronic irritability** and frequent **severe temper outbursts** that are disproportionate to the situation.
- The disorder was introduced in the DSM-5 to address concerns about the over-diagnosis of **pediatric bipolar disorder**.
- These outbursts occur at least **three times per week**, and irritability is present between outbursts.

Impact:

Depressive disorders can interfere with a child's ability to **function socially**, **academically**, and within the family. **Psychotherapy** (e.g., **CBT**) is often the first-line treatment, and **antidepressant medications** (e.g., **SSRIs**) may be considered in moderate to severe cases.

14.1.4. Autism Spectrum Disorder (ASD)

Autism Spectrum Disorder (ASD) is a neurodevelopmental disorder that affects **communication**, **social interaction**, and **behavior**. The symptoms of ASD are variable, and children with the disorder can range from highly functional to severely impaired.

Core Symptoms:

- **Social Communication Deficits**:
  - Difficulty with **eye contact**, understanding **social cues**, and engaging in **reciprocal interactions**.
  - Challenges in **developing relationships** with peers and caregivers.
- **Repetitive Behaviors**:
  - **Restricted interests**, **insistence on sameness**, and **repetitive movements** (e.g., hand flapping, rocking).

- **Sensory sensitivities**, such as overreaction to sounds, textures, or lights.

Comorbidities:

- Children with ASD may also have:
    - **Intellectual disability**
    - **ADHD**
    - **Anxiety disorders**

Impact:

ASD significantly affects a child's ability to interact socially and engage in normal developmental activities. Early **intervention programs** that focus on **behavioral therapies** and **communication skills** are critical for improving outcomes.

14.1.5. Oppositional Defiant Disorder (ODD) and Conduct Disorder

Oppositional Defiant Disorder (ODD):

- ODD is characterized by a pattern of **angry/irritable mood**, **argumentative/defiant behavior**, and **vindictiveness** toward authority figures, lasting at least **six months**.
- Symptoms include:
    - Frequent **temper tantrums**.
    - Refusal to comply with **rules** or **requests**.
    - **Blaming others** for one's own mistakes or behavior.

Conduct Disorder:

- **Conduct Disorder** involves more severe behavior problems, including **aggression** toward people or animals, **destruction of property**, **theft**, and **violations of social norms**.
- Children with **conduct disorder** are at higher risk of developing **antisocial personality disorder** in adulthood.

Impact:

Both ODD and Conduct Disorder can lead to **school problems**, difficulties with **authority figures**, and **social isolation**. Early intervention, often involving **parent management training**, **cognitive-behavioral therapy (CBT)**, and in some cases **medication**, is essential for managing symptoms and preventing escalation.

14.2. Pharmacotherapy Considerations and Evidence-Based Treatments in Pediatric Psychiatry

The management of psychiatric disorders in children and adolescents often involves a combination of **pharmacotherapy** and **evidence-based psychotherapeutic approaches**.

Treatment decisions must consider developmental stages, the unique side effect profiles of medications in younger populations, and the necessity of engaging both children and their families in therapeutic interventions.

14.2.1. Attention-Deficit/Hyperactivity Disorder (ADHD)

ADHD is one of the most commonly diagnosed psychiatric disorders in children, characterized by inattention, hyperactivity, and impulsivity. **Pharmacotherapy** is a cornerstone of ADHD management, particularly for children with moderate to severe symptoms.

Stimulants:

- **Methylphenidate-based** stimulants (e.g., **Ritalin, Concerta**) and **amphetamine-based** stimulants (e.g., **Adderall, Vyvanse**) are the **first-line treatments** for ADHD. These medications work by increasing **dopamine** and **norepinephrine** levels in the **prefrontal cortex**, improving **attention, impulse control,** and **executive functioning**.
- **Efficacy**: Stimulants have been shown to be highly effective in reducing core ADHD symptoms, with response rates as high as **70-80%** in children.
- **Side Effects**: Common side effects include **decreased appetite, insomnia, headaches,** and **mood swings**. Growth suppression has been observed in some cases, though this effect is typically mild and may normalize over time.
- **Monitoring**: Close monitoring of **height, weight,** and **sleep** is essential during stimulant treatment, and adjustments may be required based on side effects or treatment response.

Non-Stimulants:

- **Atomoxetine (Strattera)**: A **selective norepinephrine reuptake inhibitor (NRI)**, Atomoxetine is an alternative to stimulants, particularly for children who experience side effects or have a **history of substance abuse**.
    - **Efficacy**: Atomoxetine is effective, though it has a slower onset of action compared to stimulants, often taking several weeks to show full benefits.
    - **Side Effects**: It may cause **nausea, fatigue,** and **decreased appetite**, but has a lower risk of **insomnia** compared to stimulants.
- **Alpha-2 Adrenergic Agonists** (e.g., **guanfacine, clonidine**): These medications are often used in combination with stimulants or alone in cases where **tics** or **aggressive behaviors** are present.
    - **Efficacy**: They are particularly useful for managing **hyperactivity** and **impulsivity**.
    - **Side Effects**: Common side effects include **drowsiness, hypotension,** and **dry mouth**.

14.2.2. Anxiety and Depression

Anxiety and **depressive disorders** are prevalent in pediatric populations and can significantly impact functioning across social, academic, and family domains. **Pharmacotherapy** combined with **psychotherapy** is often recommended for moderate to severe cases.

Selective Serotonin Reuptake Inhibitors (SSRIs):

- **SSRIs**, such as **fluoxetine** (Prozac) and **sertraline** (Zoloft), are **first-line pharmacological treatments** for pediatric anxiety and depression.
    - **Mechanism**: SSRIs work by increasing **serotonin** levels in the brain, which improves **mood** and reduces **anxiety**.
    - **Efficacy**: Fluoxetine is FDA-approved for **major depressive disorder (MDD)** in children aged **8 years and older** and for **obsessive-compulsive disorder (OCD)**. SSRIs have demonstrated efficacy in **generalized anxiety disorder (GAD)**, **social anxiety disorder**, and **separation anxiety disorder**.
    - **Side Effects**: SSRIs are generally well-tolerated but carry a **black box warning** for increased risk of **suicidal thoughts** in children and adolescents, especially during the first few weeks of treatment.
    - **Monitoring**: Regular follow-ups are critical during the initial stages of SSRI treatment to monitor for **mood changes**, **irritability**, and **suicidal ideation**.

Cognitive Behavioral Therapy (CBT):

- **CBT** is a **gold-standard psychotherapeutic approach** for treating both **anxiety** and **depression** in children and adolescents.
    - **Focus**: CBT helps children **identify negative thought patterns**, **challenge cognitive distortions**, and **develop coping skills** to manage symptoms of anxiety and depression.
    - **Efficacy**: CBT has been shown to significantly improve functioning and symptom severity, often used as a **first-line treatment** or in combination with **pharmacotherapy** for more severe cases.

14.2.3. Autism Spectrum Disorder (ASD)

Autism Spectrum Disorder (ASD) is a **neurodevelopmental disorder** characterized by challenges in **social communication** and **restricted repetitive behaviors**. Pharmacotherapy does not address the core symptoms of ASD but can be beneficial for managing **comorbid conditions** such as **irritability**, **aggression**, and **self-injurious behaviors**.

Behavioral Interventions:

- **Early Intensive Behavioral Intervention (EIBI)** and **Applied Behavior Analysis (ABA)** are **evidence-based therapies** aimed at improving **communication**, **social skills**, and **adaptive behaviors**.
    - **Efficacy**: These interventions are most effective when started early in life and involve **structured teaching** across various developmental domains.

Medications:

- **Risperidone** and **aripiprazole** are **FDA-approved** for treating **irritability** associated with ASD in children aged **5 and older**.
    - **Mechanism**: These **atypical antipsychotics** target **dopamine** and **serotonin receptors** and are effective in reducing **aggression**, **self-injurious behaviors**, and **severe tantrums**.
    - **Side Effects**: The most common side effects include **weight gain**, **sedation**, and **metabolic syndrome** (e.g., increased risk of **diabetes**, **dyslipidemia**), necessitating close monitoring of **weight**, **glucose**, and **lipid levels** during treatment.

14.2.4. Oppositional Defiant Disorder (ODD) and Conduct Disorder

ODD and **Conduct Disorder** are disruptive behavior disorders that involve patterns of **defiant**, **argumentative**, and **aggressive behaviors**. Treatment is typically multimodal, involving **behavioral interventions** and, when necessary, pharmacotherapy for **comorbid conditions**.

Parent Management Training (PMT):

- **PMT** is an **evidence-based intervention** where parents are trained to reinforce **positive behaviors** and reduce **negative behaviors** through structured strategies.
    - **Efficacy**: PMT has been shown to reduce the severity of ODD symptoms by teaching parents **consistency** in discipline, **positive reinforcement**, and effective communication skills.

Multisystemic Therapy (MST):

- **MST** is an intensive family- and community-based intervention aimed at reducing **delinquent behavior** in adolescents with **Conduct Disorder**.
    - **Efficacy**: MST focuses on the child's **family**, **school**, and **peer group**, providing a holistic approach to reducing **antisocial behavior** and improving **family dynamics**.

Medications:

- While no specific medications target ODD or Conduct Disorder, pharmacotherapy may be used to treat **comorbid conditions** such as **ADHD**, **depression**, or **bipolar disorder**.
    - **Stimulants**: For children with **ADHD** and **ODD**, stimulants like **methylphenidate** may help reduce **hyperactivity** and **impulsivity**.
    - **SSRIs**: For children with **comorbid depression** or **anxiety**, SSRIs may be used to manage mood symptoms.
    - **Mood Stabilizers** (e.g., **valproate**, **lithium**) may be used for children with **severe mood dysregulation** or **aggressive behaviors** associated with conduct disorder.

14.3. Monitoring for Adverse Effects and Optimizing Medication Regimens in Pediatric Patients

Managing psychiatric conditions in pediatric patients requires a careful balance between efficacy and safety due to their developing bodies and brains. **Psychotropic medications** can provide significant benefits, but regular and careful **monitoring** is crucial to minimize the risk of adverse effects. Optimizing medication regimens involves starting with the lowest effective dose, avoiding unnecessary polypharmacy, and tapering medications when appropriate.

14.3.1. Monitoring for Adverse Effects

Pediatric patients are particularly vulnerable to the side effects of psychotropic medications, which can affect growth, development, and overall well-being. Regular monitoring not only helps in detecting adverse effects early but also ensures the treatment remains appropriate as the child grows.

Stimulants (ADHD Medications)

- **Common Medications**: Methylphenidate (e.g., **Ritalin**, **Concerta**), amphetamine-based stimulants (e.g., **Adderall**, **Vyvanse**).
- **Potential Adverse Effects**:
  - **Growth Suppression**: **Decreased appetite** is a common side effect, potentially leading to **reduced caloric intake** and slower **physical growth**. This is particularly concerning in younger children who are still in crucial stages of development.
  - **Sleep Disturbances**: Many children experience **insomnia** or difficulty falling asleep due to the stimulant's effects.
  - **Mood Changes**: Irritability, increased **anxiety**, or **mood swings** may occur, especially as the medication wears off at the end of the day.
- **Monitoring Guidelines**:
  - **Height and weight** should be tracked regularly, with measurements ideally taken at every follow-up visit. This helps detect any trends in slowed growth or weight loss.
  - **Vital signs** (heart rate, blood pressure) should be checked periodically to ensure the medication does not cause excessive **tachycardia** or **hypertension**.
  - **Sleep patterns** and **appetite** should be discussed at every visit, with parents encouraged to track changes at home. Adjusting the dosing schedule or the type of stimulant (short-acting vs. long-acting) may help mitigate these issues.

Selective Serotonin Reuptake Inhibitors (SSRIs)

SSRIs are often used to treat **anxiety** and **depressive disorders** in children, but they carry particular risks that require close monitoring.

- **Common Medications**: Fluoxetine (Prozac), Sertraline (Zoloft).
- **Potential Adverse Effects**:
    - **Suicidal Thoughts**: The **black box warning** for SSRIs highlights the increased risk of **suicidal ideation** and behaviors in children, especially during the first few weeks of treatment or after dose adjustments.
    - **Activation Syndrome**: Children may experience **increased restlessness**, **hyperactivity**, or **agitation** when starting an SSRI, which can mimic **mania** or **bipolar disorder**.
    - **Mood Changes**: Increased **irritability**, **impulsivity**, or **emotional lability** should be monitored closely, as these may indicate an inappropriate dose or the need for a different therapeutic approach.
- **Monitoring Guidelines**:
    - Close **follow-up appointments** should be scheduled in the initial stages of SSRI treatment, typically within the first **1-2 weeks**, and then monthly to assess for changes in **mood**, **behavior**, and **suicidal ideation**.
    - Parents and caregivers should be educated about potential warning signs, such as **sudden changes in behavior**, **withdrawal**, or **increased aggression**, and should report these symptoms immediately.
    - Ongoing monitoring of **sleep**, **appetite**, and **energy levels** is also necessary to evaluate the balance between therapeutic benefits and side effects.

Atypical Antipsychotics

Atypical antipsychotics, such as **risperidone** and **aripiprazole**, are commonly used to manage **irritability**, **aggression**, and **mood disorders** in pediatric patients, especially those with **autism spectrum disorder (ASD)** or **bipolar disorder**. However, they carry significant risks for **metabolic side effects**.

- **Common Medications**: Risperidone (Risperdal), Aripiprazole (Abilify).
- **Potential Adverse Effects**:
    - **Weight Gain**: Atypical antipsychotics are associated with significant **weight gain**, which can predispose children to **obesity** and related health conditions.
    - **Metabolic Syndrome**: Children may develop **hyperglycemia**, **insulin resistance**, or **dyslipidemia** (elevated cholesterol and triglycerides), increasing the risk of **diabetes**.
    - **Sedation**: Excessive **drowsiness** or **fatigue** may affect school performance and social engagement.
- **Monitoring Guidelines**:
    - **Body Mass Index (BMI)** should be tracked regularly to monitor for excessive weight gain. This is typically assessed every **3-6 months**, depending on the individual's risk factors.
    - **Blood glucose levels** and **lipid profiles** should be tested at baseline and periodically throughout treatment to detect early signs of **metabolic syndrome**.
    - Parents should be encouraged to promote **healthy eating habits** and regular **physical activity** to help mitigate weight gain.

14.3.2. Optimizing Medication Regimens

In pediatric psychiatry, optimizing medication regimens involves using the lowest effective dose, minimizing the risk of drug interactions, and considering the child's developmental stage and individual needs. The goal is to provide therapeutic benefits while reducing the potential for side effects.

Starting Low and Going Slow:

- Medications should be started at **low doses**, especially in younger children, and **titrated slowly** based on the child's response and side effects.
    - For example, starting with the lowest available dose of a stimulant for **ADHD** or a **SSRI** for anxiety allows the clinician to adjust upward as needed while monitoring for adverse effects.
    - **Slow titration** also reduces the risk of **activation syndrome** or **increased irritability**, which can be more common with rapid dose escalation.

Avoiding Polypharmacy:

- **Polypharmacy** (the use of multiple medications) should be avoided when possible. Combining multiple psychotropic medications increases the risk of **drug interactions**, **compounded side effects**, and **non-adherence**.
    - When a child presents with **multiple comorbid conditions** (e.g., ADHD and anxiety), clinicians should consider **monotherapy** first before adding additional medications.
    - Regular **medication reviews** should be conducted to assess whether all prescribed medications are necessary and to avoid duplications of therapeutic effects.

Tapering and Discontinuation:

- For children who have shown **significant improvement**, it may be appropriate to consider **tapering** medications to minimize the long-term impact of psychotropic drugs. However, this should be done cautiously.
    - **ADHD medications**: Children may be tapered off during **school vacations** or breaks to assess whether they continue to require the medication.
    - **SSRIs for anxiety or depression**: **Gradual tapering** over weeks or months is necessary to prevent **withdrawal symptoms** and avoid **relapse** of the original condition.
- **Close supervision** is required during tapering to monitor for any return of symptoms. If symptoms re-emerge, re-initiation of treatment at a lower dose or a more prolonged tapering plan may be necessary.

14.4. Role of Advanced Pharmacist Practitioners in Pediatric Mental Health Care

Pharmacist practitioners play a crucial role in pediatric mental health care by ensuring safe and effective medication management, providing patient and caregiver education, and collaborating with other healthcare providers to optimize treatment outcomes.

14.4.1. Medication Counseling:

Pharmacist practitioners provide education to parents and caregivers on the **proper use of medications**, potential side effects, and the importance of adherence to prescribed treatments. They can explain the rationale behind medication choices and address concerns about the long-term use of psychotropic medications in children.

14.4.2. Monitoring and Management of Adverse Effects:

Pharmacists are responsible for monitoring medication safety and efficacy, ensuring that children are not experiencing significant adverse effects. They can assist in the **adjustment of doses** or recommend alternative therapies if side effects become problematic.

14.4.3. Collaborative Care:

Pharmacists work closely with **pediatricians**, **psychiatrists**, and **therapists** to provide integrated care for children with psychiatric disorders. This collaborative approach ensures that treatment plans are tailored to the individual needs of the child and that all aspects of care, including **behavioral therapies** and **school accommodations**, are coordinated.

14.4.4. Addressing Polypharmacy:

Pharmacists are well-positioned to identify cases of **polypharmacy**, where children may be on multiple psychotropic or non-psychotropic medications. They can work with prescribers to simplify medication regimens and minimize drug interactions, especially in children with complex psychiatric and medical conditions.

Pediatric psychiatric disorders require careful diagnosis and management, with a combination of **pharmacotherapy** and **behavioral interventions** playing a critical role in treatment. Stimulants, SSRIs, and atypical antipsychotics are commonly used but require close monitoring for adverse effects in children.

Advanced pharmacist practitioners are integral to ensuring the safe and effective use of medications, providing education to families, and collaborating with healthcare providers to optimize treatment outcomes. Early intervention and a comprehensive, multidisciplinary approach are essential to improving the mental health and well-being of children and adolescents.

References:

1. American Psychiatric Association. (2013). *Diagnostic and Statistical Manual of Mental Disorders* (5th ed.).
2. Pliszka, S. R. (2007). Practice parameter for the assessment and treatment of children and adolescents with attention-deficit/hyperactivity disorder. *Journal of the American Academy of Child & Adolescent Psychiatry*, 46(7), 894-921.
3. McClellan, J., Stock, S., & American Academy of Child and Adolescent Psychiatry (AACAP). (2013). Practice parameter for the assessment and treatment of children and adolescents with schizophrenia. *Journal of the American Academy of Child & Adolescent Psychiatry*, 52(9), 976-990.
4. Vitiello, B., & Towbin, K. (2018). Pharmacologic treatment of child and adolescent psychiatric disorders. *Journal of Child Psychology and Psychiatry*, 59(2), 119-124.
5. Ghuman, J. K., & Ghuman, H. S. (2013). Pharmacological treatment of anxiety disorders in children and adolescents. *Journal of Clinical Psychiatry*, 74(6), e620-e628.
6. Volkmar, F. R., Siegel, M., Woodbury-Smith, M., et al. (2014). Practice parameter for the assessment and treatment of children and adolescents with autism spectrum disorder. *Journal of the American Academy of Child & Adolescent Psychiatry*, 53(2), 237-257.

Chapter 15: Cultural Competence and Psychiatric Care

Cultural competence is critical in psychiatric care, as cultural beliefs, values, and practices significantly influence how individuals perceive mental health, seek treatment, and respond to interventions. Addressing these cultural factors can improve the quality of care and promote equity for diverse patient populations.

This chapter will explore the importance of **understanding cultural influences on mental health beliefs and practices**, strategies for **providing culturally competent care**, and approaches to **addressing health disparities and promoting equity** in psychiatric care delivery.

15.1. Understanding Cultural Influences on Mental Health Beliefs and Practices

Cultural influences significantly shape how individuals perceive mental health, experience psychiatric symptoms, and seek treatment. Understanding these influences is essential for healthcare providers to deliver culturally sensitive and effective care. Mental health is deeply intertwined with cultural norms, religious beliefs, and societal values, all of which can impact a person's willingness to seek help, adhere to treatment, and express symptoms. Below is an elaboration on the ways in which culture affects mental health beliefs and practices, with examples from different cultural contexts.

15.1.1. Cultural Perceptions of Mental Health

Each culture has its own perspective on mental health, illness, and the nature of psychiatric symptoms. These cultural views influence how individuals and communities recognize mental health problems and whether they seek professional treatment.

Stigma and Mental Health

In many cultures, **mental illness** is associated with significant **stigma**, which can prevent individuals from seeking help due to fear of **judgment**, **shame**, or **social exclusion**.

- **Example 1: Stigma in Asian Cultures**: In many **Asian cultures**, mental illness is often viewed as a **weakness** or a **failure** of self-control, which can bring shame not only to the individual but also to their family. For instance, in **Chinese** and **Japanese** societies, individuals may avoid disclosing mental health issues or seeking treatment to protect the family's **social standing**. As a result, psychiatric conditions like **depression** may go untreated, and individuals may instead focus on **physical symptoms** (e.g., **headaches**, **fatigue**) as a socially acceptable way to express distress.
- **Example 2: Mental Health in Middle Eastern Cultures**: In some **Middle Eastern cultures**, mental illness may be seen as a **disgrace** or a punishment for moral or religious failings. This stigma can prevent people from accessing psychiatric services or

may push them toward alternative treatments, such as **spiritual healing** or **religious counsel**. For instance, in some communities, **depression** may be viewed as a spiritual weakness, leading individuals to seek help from **religious leaders** or **traditional healers** rather than mental health professionals.

Spiritual and Religious Beliefs

In many cultures, **mental health issues** are often understood through a **spiritual** or **religious lens**, which can lead individuals to attribute psychiatric symptoms to **supernatural** causes. In such cases, people may prioritize spiritual remedies over professional psychiatric care.

- **Example 3: Supernatural Explanations in African Cultures**: In some **African cultures**, mental health problems such as **psychosis** may be attributed to **spirit possession** or **curses**. For example, in parts of **West Africa**, mental illness is sometimes seen as the result of **witchcraft** or **evil spirits**. This belief may lead individuals to seek help from **traditional healers** or engage in **rituals** and **exorcisms** to remove the supernatural cause, rather than accessing psychiatric treatment.
- **Example 4: Religious Interpretations in South Asian Cultures**: In **India**, some individuals may attribute **mental health symptoms** to **divine punishment** or **karma**. For instance, a person experiencing **depression** or **anxiety** might believe they are being punished for past actions in a previous life. As a result, they may turn to **prayers**, **pilgrimages**, or **religious ceremonies** to seek relief, delaying or avoiding mental health treatment altogether.

15.1.2. Culture-Bound Syndromes

Certain psychiatric symptoms and syndromes are unique to specific cultural contexts and are shaped by **local beliefs**, **traditions**, and **environmental factors**. These **culture-bound syndromes** highlight how cultural frameworks shape the expression of mental distress.

Examples of Culture-Bound Syndromes:

- **Example 5: Ataque de Nervios**:
  - This syndrome is primarily found in **Latin American cultures** and is characterized by episodes of intense emotional distress, including **crying**, **screaming**, and sometimes **physical aggression**. It often occurs in response to **stressful events** such as family conflict or the death of a loved one. Individuals experiencing **Ataque de Nervios** may attribute their symptoms to a temporary loss of control and seek support from family and **spiritual leaders** rather than psychiatric professionals.
- **Example 6: Kufungisisa (Thinking Too Much)**:
  - In **Zimbabwe**, **Kufungisisa** is a cultural syndrome that translates to "thinking too much" and is associated with symptoms of **anxiety** and **depression**. Individuals who suffer from **Kufungisisa** experience **ruminative thoughts** about life difficulties, which are viewed as a cause of physical and emotional distress. The

cultural understanding of **Kufungisisa** often leads individuals to seek support from **traditional healers** or **herbalists**.
- **Example 7: Dhat Syndrome**:
  - **Dhat Syndrome** is commonly found in **South Asia**, particularly among **Indian** men. It involves **extreme anxiety** about the loss of **semen**, which is culturally viewed as a vital life force. Men with **Dhat Syndrome** report symptoms like **fatigue, weakness, depression,** and **sexual dysfunction**. Because of cultural beliefs about the importance of semen, affected individuals may seek remedies from **Ayurvedic** or **Unani** healers rather than modern psychiatric care.

15.1.3. Cultural Influences on Treatment Preferences

Cultural beliefs also shape preferences for certain types of treatment over others. In some cultures, traditional healing practices or holistic approaches are preferred over conventional psychiatric treatments. Moreover, the involvement of family in decision-making varies significantly between cultures.

Holistic and Traditional Healers:

- **Example 8: Traditional Healing in Indigenous Cultures**: In many **Indigenous cultures**, mental health is viewed in a holistic way, connected to **spirituality, nature,** and the community. For instance, some **Native American** tribes rely on **medicine men** or **shamans** to provide **healing ceremonies** that address mental, physical, and spiritual imbalances. These traditional healers may use a combination of **herbal remedies, rituals,** and **storytelling** to address psychiatric symptoms. Modern psychiatric interventions may be seen as secondary or less culturally appropriate.
- **Example 9: Herbal Remedies in Chinese Medicine**: In **Traditional Chinese Medicine (TCM)**, mental health issues such as **anxiety** or **depression** are often understood as imbalances in the body's **qi** (vital energy). Patients may prefer **herbal remedies, acupuncture,** or **qigong** (a practice combining movement, meditation, and breath control) over Western psychiatric treatments like **SSRIs** or **cognitive behavioral therapy (CBT)**.

Family Involvement in Treatment:

- **Example 10: Collectivist Cultures**: In many **Asian** and **Latin American cultures**, family involvement is central to healthcare decisions. In **Chinese** or **Mexican** families, decisions about mental health treatment may involve not only the patient but also **extended family members**. The family's well-being and values are often prioritized over individual autonomy, meaning that treatment options may be chosen based on what is best for the family unit as a whole. This cultural perspective can impact how mental health services are delivered and how information is shared with patients and families.
- **Example 11: Individualistic Cultures**: In contrast, **Western** cultures, such as the **United States** or **Europe**, typically emphasize **individual autonomy**. Patients are expected to make their own decisions about mental health treatment, even if it conflicts

with family preferences. This individualistic approach can create challenges when working with patients from more **collectivist** backgrounds, where family involvement is deeply embedded in healthcare practices.

15.2. Providing Culturally Competent Care to Diverse Patient Populations

Culturally competent care involves recognizing, respecting, and integrating patients' cultural backgrounds into psychiatric care. It also requires an understanding of how cultural factors influence mental health and treatment outcomes.

15.2.1. Cultural Assessment in Psychiatric Evaluation:

Conducting a **cultural assessment** as part of the psychiatric evaluation is essential for understanding the patient's worldview, beliefs about mental health, and preferences for treatment. The **DSM-5** includes a **Cultural Formulation Interview (CFI)**, a structured tool that helps clinicians explore the patient's cultural identity, the cultural meaning of their symptoms, and their cultural expectations for care.

Key components of a cultural assessment include:

- **Cultural Identity**: Understanding the patient's cultural background, language preferences, and degree of acculturation or assimilation into the dominant culture.
- **Cultural Explanations of Illness**: Exploring the patient's beliefs about the cause of their symptoms, whether they attribute their condition to biological, psychological, or spiritual factors.
- **Cultural Factors in Coping and Help-Seeking**: Assessing how the patient and their family have coped with symptoms in the past and what types of help they are open to receiving (e.g., spiritual healers, family support, professional treatment).
- **Language and Communication**: Ensuring that language barriers are addressed through the use of **qualified interpreters** or bilingual mental health professionals, rather than relying on family members or untrained individuals.

15.2.2. Culturally Adapted Psychotherapy:

Adapting psychotherapeutic approaches to align with the patient's cultural background can enhance the therapeutic alliance and improve outcomes. Culturally adapted psychotherapy takes into account the patient's worldview, values, and communication styles.

- **Cognitive Behavioral Therapy (CBT)**: CBT can be adapted to different cultural contexts by incorporating culturally relevant metaphors, addressing culturally specific beliefs (e.g., fatalism, collectivism), and involving family members when appropriate. For example, in some Asian cultures, CBT may focus on **interpersonal harmony** and **family obligations** rather than individual self-assertion.
- **Narrative Therapy**: This approach encourages patients to reframe their experiences through storytelling, which can be particularly effective in cultures that value oral traditions or collective memory.

- **Trauma-Informed Care**: In refugee and immigrant populations, trauma-informed care is essential, as many individuals may have experienced war, displacement, or violence. This approach prioritizes safety, trust, and empowerment, recognizing the impact of trauma on mental health.

15.2.3. Cultural Competence Training for Clinicians:

Ongoing **cultural competence training** for mental health professionals is essential for delivering culturally responsive care. This training should include:

- **Self-Reflection**: Encouraging clinicians to reflect on their own cultural biases, assumptions, and potential blind spots.
- **Cultural Humility**: Fostering an attitude of openness and willingness to learn from patients about their cultural background and perspectives.
- **Cross-Cultural Communication**: Developing skills for effective communication across cultural and linguistic differences, including the use of interpreters and culturally sensitive language.

15.3. Addressing Health Disparities and Promoting Equity in Psychiatric Care Delivery

15.3.1. Health Disparities in Mental Health Care:

Health disparities refer to differences in the quality of care and health outcomes between different populations, often based on race, ethnicity, socioeconomic status, or geographic location. In psychiatric care, **racial and ethnic minorities**, **immigrants**, and **low-income populations** are more likely to experience barriers to accessing mental health services, lower quality of care, and worse outcomes.

- **Access to Care**: Minority populations often face structural barriers to accessing mental health care, including lack of insurance, geographic isolation, and a shortage of mental health professionals in underserved areas.
- **Disparities in Diagnosis and Treatment**: Racial and ethnic minorities are less likely to receive a timely diagnosis of mental health conditions and more likely to be diagnosed with **severe psychiatric conditions** (e.g., **schizophrenia**) rather than **mood disorders**. They are also less likely to receive **evidence-based treatments**, such as psychotherapy or appropriate psychotropic medications.
- **Cultural Mistrust**: Historical injustices and discrimination in the healthcare system have contributed to **mistrust** of medical institutions among minority groups, particularly African Americans and Indigenous populations. This mistrust can lead to delays in seeking care or reluctance to engage with treatment.

15.3.2. Promoting Equity in Psychiatric Care:

To address health disparities and promote equity in psychiatric care, healthcare systems and providers must focus on creating **inclusive, accessible**, and **culturally responsive** services.

- **Community Engagement**: Partnering with community leaders, religious organizations, and cultural groups can help bridge the gap between healthcare providers and underserved populations. **Community mental health workers** and **peer support specialists** from similar cultural backgrounds can play a crucial role in outreach and engagement.
- **Culturally Tailored Interventions**: Developing interventions that are tailored to the needs and preferences of specific cultural groups can improve treatment adherence and outcomes. For example, integrating **spiritual counseling** or **traditional healing practices** with psychiatric care may be more acceptable to certain cultural groups.
- **Addressing Structural Barriers**: Policies that improve access to mental health care, such as expanding insurance coverage, increasing the availability of **telepsychiatry** in rural areas, and ensuring **language services** in healthcare settings, are essential for reducing disparities.

15.3.3. Addressing Social Determinants of Mental Health:

Mental health disparities are closely linked to **social determinants of health**, such as **poverty, housing insecurity, education,** and **employment opportunities**. Mental health providers should be aware of these factors and advocate for policies that address the underlying social conditions contributing to poor mental health.

- **Integrated Care Models**: Integrating mental health care with **primary care** and **social services** can help address the broader social determinants of health. For example, **collaborative care models** that involve social workers, housing support, and legal aid can improve mental health outcomes for individuals experiencing homelessness or financial instability.

Cultural competence is essential in providing high-quality psychiatric care to diverse patient populations. Understanding the cultural influences on mental health beliefs and practices allows clinicians to provide care that respects the patient's worldview and preferences.

Culturally competent care, combined with efforts to address health disparities, can help promote equity and improve mental health outcomes for underserved and marginalized populations. By adopting culturally responsive approaches and addressing the social determinants of mental health, psychiatric care can become more inclusive and accessible to all.

References:

1. American Psychiatric Association. (2013). *Diagnostic and Statistical Manual of Mental Disorders* (5th ed.).
2. Sue, S., Zane, N., & Nagayama Hall, G. C. (2009). The cultural context of therapeutic intervention. In H. S. Friedman (Ed.), *The Oxford Handbook of Health Psychology* (pp. 571-590). Oxford University Press.
3. Kleinman, A. (1980). **Patients and Healers in the Context of Culture**. Berkeley, CA: University of California Press.
4. Snowden, L. R. (2001). Barriers to effective mental health services for African Americans. *Mental Health Services Research*, 3(4), 181-187.
5. Lewis-Fernández, R., & Aggarwal, N. K. (2013). Culture and psychiatric evaluation: DSM-5® Cultural Formulation Interview. *Psychiatric Clinics of North America*, 36(3), 543-560.
6. Betancourt, J. R., Green, A. R., & Carrillo, J. E. (2002). Cultural competence in health care: Emerging frameworks and practical approaches. *The Commonwealth Fund*.
7. Vega, W. A., & Rumbaut, R. G. (1991). Ethnic minorities and mental health. *Annual Review of Sociology*, 17, 351-383.

Chapter 16: Collaborative Care and Interprofessional Collaboration

Collaborative care and interprofessional collaboration are essential in managing psychiatric disorders, particularly in complex cases where multiple healthcare professionals are involved. These models foster communication, shared decision-making, and comprehensive care, ultimately improving patient outcomes. This chapter explores the **importance of collaborative care models**, the **role of pharmacist practitioners** in interdisciplinary mental health teams, strategies for **effective communication** with healthcare providers, and presents **case studies** to illustrate successful interprofessional collaboration in psychiatric care.

16.1. Importance of Collaborative Care Models in Managing Psychiatric Disorders

16.1.1. Definition and Key Components of Collaborative Care:

Collaborative care is a **team-based** approach to healthcare that integrates medical, mental health, and other care services to manage psychiatric disorders. The model emphasizes **communication** and **coordination** among healthcare providers, ensuring that treatment is comprehensive and patient-centered.

Key components of collaborative care include:

- **Interdisciplinary Teams**: Involves collaboration between mental health professionals (psychiatrists, psychologists, social workers), primary care physicians, pharmacists, and other specialists.
- **Care Coordination**: A care manager (e.g., nurse or social worker) typically helps coordinate treatment across different providers, ensuring that the patient's care plan is integrated and that all team members are informed of the patient's progress.
- **Evidence-Based Treatment**: Collaborative care uses evidence-based psychotherapies and pharmacological treatments that are tailored to the patient's needs.
- **Measurement-Based Care**: Progress is routinely monitored using standardized assessment tools (e.g., the **Patient Health Questionnaire-9** for depression), and treatment is adjusted based on the patient's response.

16.1.2. Benefits of Collaborative Care:

- **Improved Access to Mental Health Care**: Collaborative care allows for the integration of psychiatric services in **primary care settings**, making mental health care more accessible to patients who may otherwise face barriers to seeing a specialist.
- **Better Outcomes**: Studies have shown that collaborative care models are associated with better outcomes for patients with **depression**, **anxiety**, and **bipolar disorder**. These models improve symptom management, reduce hospitalizations, and enhance overall quality of life .

- **Cost-Effectiveness**: By reducing hospitalizations, emergency department visits, and overall healthcare costs, collaborative care is considered a cost-effective approach to managing psychiatric disorders.

16.1.3. Collaborative Care for Specific Populations:

- **Chronic Medical Conditions**: Collaborative care is particularly effective for individuals with **comorbid psychiatric** and **chronic medical conditions** (e.g., diabetes, heart disease). For example, patients with **diabetes** and **depression** benefit from a care model that integrates psychiatric treatment with diabetes management, addressing both physical and mental health needs simultaneously.
- **Substance Use Disorders**: Collaborative care models that integrate **addiction specialists** and mental health providers have shown success in managing co-occurring **substance use** and **psychiatric disorders**, improving both mental health and recovery outcomes.

16.2. Role of Advanced Pharmacist Practitioners in Interdisciplinary Mental Health Teams

16.2.1. Pharmacist's Role in Medication Management:

Pharmacist practitioners are essential members of the collaborative care team, especially in managing complex psychotropic medication regimens. Their role includes:

- **Medication Reconciliation**: Ensuring accuracy in the patient's medication list by reviewing prescriptions, over-the-counter medications, and supplements.
- **Optimizing Medication Regimens**: Pharmacists assess the efficacy and safety of psychotropic medications, adjusting doses, or recommending alternative treatments to minimize side effects and improve therapeutic outcomes. For example, they may recommend switching from a first-generation antipsychotic to a second-generation antipsychotic to reduce the risk of extrapyramidal side effects.
- **Monitoring for Drug Interactions**: Pharmacists identify potential **drug-drug interactions**, especially in patients on multiple medications (polypharmacy), ensuring that combinations of psychotropic and other medications (e.g., cardiovascular or diabetic medications) are safe and effective.

16.2.2. Pharmacist's Role in Patient Education and Adherence:

Pharmacists play a critical role in educating patients about their medications and ensuring adherence to treatment plans.

- **Patient Counseling**: Pharmacists provide detailed explanations about the purpose of the medication, expected benefits, potential side effects, and what to do if a dose is missed. For instance, explaining the **delayed onset** of antidepressants can help manage patient expectations and encourage adherence.

- **Adherence Support**: Pharmacists may help design strategies to improve adherence, such as simplifying dosing regimens, providing blister packs, or utilizing medication reminders for patients with cognitive impairments.

16.2.3. Collaborative Decision-Making:

Pharmacists collaborate closely with psychiatrists, primary care physicians, and other team members to develop and implement treatment plans. For example, if a patient experiences intolerable side effects from a medication, the pharmacist can recommend adjustments or alternative medications, working in tandem with the psychiatrist to make informed decisions that prioritize the patient's well-being.

16.3. Effective Communication and Collaboration with Other Healthcare Providers

16.3.1. Building a Collaborative Culture:

Successful interprofessional collaboration requires a culture of **mutual respect** and **open communication**. All team members must feel comfortable sharing their perspectives and expertise, and decision-making should be **shared** rather than hierarchical.

- **Team Meetings and Case Conferences**: Regular team meetings, case reviews, and interdisciplinary conferences provide a forum for healthcare providers to discuss patient progress, review treatment plans, and adjust care based on input from all team members.
- **Documentation and Communication Tools**: The use of **shared electronic health records (EHRs)** ensures that all providers have access to up-to-date information about the patient's treatment. Pharmacists can document medication changes, lab results, and therapeutic recommendations in the EHR, which can be reviewed by other team members.

16.3.2. Effective Communication Strategies:

- **SBAR (Situation-Background-Assessment-Recommendation)**: The **SBAR** model is a structured communication tool used to relay critical information between healthcare providers, ensuring clarity and brevity. For example, a pharmacist could use SBAR to communicate concerns about a patient's **non-adherence** to their psychiatrist, outlining the situation, relevant background information, an assessment of potential causes, and recommendations for improving adherence.
- **Interprofessional Rounds**: Participating in **interprofessional rounds** on inpatient psychiatric units allows pharmacists, nurses, social workers, and psychiatrists to collaborate in real-time, providing input on medication management, psychosocial interventions, and discharge planning.

16.3.3. Collaborating with Primary Care Providers:

Primary care physicians (PCPs) play a central role in the management of many patients with psychiatric disorders, especially in settings where access to psychiatrists is limited. Collaborative care models allow mental health specialists and pharmacists to work closely with PCPs, providing support for medication management and psychotherapeutic interventions.

- **Consultation and Referral**: Pharmacists can serve as a resource for PCPs who may need guidance on psychotropic medications, offering recommendations on **titration**, **side effect management**, or **medication switches** for complex patients.

16.4. Case Studies and Practical Examples of Interprofessional Collaboration in Psychiatric Care

Interprofessional collaboration in psychiatric care involves the coordinated efforts of professionals from various disciplines—such as psychiatry, psychology, nursing, social work, and pharmacology—working together to provide comprehensive care to patients with mental health conditions. Below are five case studies and practical examples that highlight the importance of interprofessional collaboration in psychiatric care.

16.4.1. Bipolar Case Study: Collaborative Management

Patient Background: A 25-year-old Chinese male patient diagnosed with **bipolar disorder** presents with frequent mood swings, non-adherence to medication, and a history of substance abuse. He has been hospitalized multiple times for manic episodes and has difficulty maintaining employment.

Interprofessional Collaboration:

- **Psychiatrist**: The lead clinician monitors the patient's medication regimen, adjusting the dosage of **mood stabilizers** (e.g., lithium) and **antipsychotics** (e.g., quetiapine) to manage manic and depressive episodes.
- **Psychologist**: Provides **Cognitive Behavioral Therapy (CBT)** to help the patient develop coping mechanisms for mood instability and identify triggers for manic episodes.
- **Social Worker**: Assists in coordinating **community resources**, including housing and employment services, to stabilize the patient's external environment and reduce stressors.
- **Substance Abuse Counselor**: Addresses the patient's **substance use** through **motivational interviewing** and relapse prevention strategies, integrating care with the psychiatric team.
- **Pharmacist**: Monitors potential **drug interactions** between the patient's psychiatric medications and any substances used, ensuring safe administration of mood stabilizers and antipsychotics.

Outcome:

Through the collaborative efforts of the care team, the patient achieves **stabilized mood** and improves **medication adherence**. Regular monitoring of the patient's mental health and substance use continues through outpatient services, reducing the risk of further hospitalizations.

16.4.2. Depression and Anxiety Case Study: Treatment of Adolescent in a School Setting

Patient Background: A 15-year-old Hispanic female student exhibits signs of **depression** and **anxiety**, including poor academic performance, social withdrawal, and frequent absences from school. Her teachers and parents are concerned about her well-being.

Interprofessional Collaboration:

- **School Psychologist**: Conducts an initial evaluation and provides short-term **counseling** and **support** to the student within the school setting, helping her identify stressors and coping strategies.
- **Pediatric Psychiatrist**: Prescribes an **SSRI** (e.g., fluoxetine) for the treatment of depression and anxiety, monitors side effects, and coordinates with the school to monitor progress.
- **School Counselor**: Works with the student to address **academic challenges** and provides strategies for **time management** and **study skills**.
- **Family Therapist**: Engages the family in therapy sessions to address **family dynamics** and **parenting strategies**, fostering a supportive home environment for the student.
- **Nurse Practitioner**: Monitors the student's physical health, particularly side effects of the SSRI, and provides **nutrition counseling** to address issues related to appetite and weight.

Outcome:

With the combined efforts of the school psychologist, psychiatrist, and other professionals, the student shows significant improvement in her **academic performance**, **social interactions**, and overall **mental health**. Continued follow-ups help ensure sustained progress and medication efficacy.

16.4.3. PTSD Case Study: Management of Post-Traumatic Stress Disorder in a Veteran

Patient Background: A 40-year-old African male veteran presents with **PTSD**, experiencing frequent **nightmares**, **flashbacks**, and **hypervigilance** following combat exposure. He also has symptoms of **depression** and **alcohol misuse**.

Interprofessional Collaboration:

- **Veterans Affairs (VA) Psychiatrist**: Prescribed **SSRIs** (e.g., sertraline) to manage PTSD symptoms and **prazosin** to reduce nightmares. Regularly assesses the patient's response to medication and adjusts the treatment plan as needed.
- **Trauma Therapist**: Provides **Trauma-Focused Cognitive Behavioral Therapy (TF-CBT)** to address the underlying trauma and teach **coping mechanisms** for distressing thoughts and flashbacks.
- **Occupational Therapist**: Helps the patient reintegrate into civilian life by focusing on building **daily routines**, managing stress, and **returning to work**.
- **Substance Abuse Counselor**: Provides treatment for **alcohol misuse**, using **motivational interviewing** and **12-step programs** to encourage sobriety.
- **Peer Support Specialist**: A fellow veteran with lived experience of PTSD offers **peer counseling**, providing emotional support and helping the patient navigate mental health resources available through the VA.

Outcome:

The patient experiences a reduction in **PTSD symptoms**, maintains **sobriety**, and successfully reintegrated into his community with improved **occupational functioning** and **social support**. Regular follow-up care ensures that both mental health and substance use issues remain under control.

16.4.4. Schizophrenia Case Study: Integrated Care in a Community Mental Health Center

Patient Background: A 30-year-old Filipino woman with **schizophrenia** presents with **delusions** and **hallucinations**, leading to severe isolation and difficulty functioning in daily life. She has poor medication adherence and limited social support.

Interprofessional Collaboration:

- **Psychiatrist**: Manages the patient's **antipsychotic** medication regimen, prescribing **risperidone** and monitoring for **side effects** such as weight gain or metabolic syndrome.
- **Community Psychiatric Nurse**: Provides in-home visits to ensure the patient takes her medication regularly, monitors for side effects, and supports daily functioning.
- **Case Manager**: Connects the patient with **housing** and **social services**, providing a stable living environment and assisting with basic needs such as transportation and grocery shopping.
- **Social Worker**: Coordinates the patient's involvement in a **community reintegration program** that helps her build **social skills** and **develop relationships** within the community.
- **Occupational Therapist**: Assists the patient with developing **independent living skills**, including managing finances, cooking, and engaging in meaningful leisure activities.

Outcome:

Through comprehensive interprofessional collaboration, the patient demonstrates **improved adherence** to her medication regimen, reduced psychotic symptoms, and an increased ability to engage in **daily activities**. Regular check-ins with the team help maintain her progress and reduce the likelihood of relapse.

16.4.5. Psychiatric Crisis Case Study: Emergency Response

Patient Background: A 22-year-old Vietnamese male with a history of **bipolar disorder** and **substance abuse** is brought to the emergency department after a suicide attempt. He is agitated, disoriented, and uncooperative, making it difficult for staff to assess him.

Interprofessional Collaboration:

- **Emergency Psychiatrist**: Leads the initial **psychiatric evaluation**, working to stabilize the patient and determine whether involuntary hospitalization is necessary. They coordinate the immediate care plan with the ED team.
- **Emergency Room Nurse**: Provides medical care, administers sedatives as necessary, and monitors the patient's vital signs to ensure safety during the initial crisis period.
- **Crisis Intervention Specialist**: Engages with the patient to de-escalate the situation, assess **suicidality**, and offer **supportive counseling** while the patient is being stabilized.
- **Substance Abuse Counselor**: Evaluates the patient for co-occurring **substance use** issues and helps develop a plan for treatment, including the possibility of a **detoxification** program after stabilization.
- **Social Worker**: Works with the family to provide support, gather collateral information, and plan for **discharge** or **transfer** to a psychiatric unit, coordinating outpatient follow-up care and connecting the patient with community resources.

Outcome:

The patient is stabilized, transferred to an inpatient psychiatric unit for further treatment, and later referred to a comprehensive **outpatient care plan** that includes psychiatric support, substance abuse treatment, and family therapy. The **crisis intervention team** successfully de-escalates the situation and ensures a smooth transition from emergency care to long-term support.

Collaborative care models and interprofessional collaboration are essential for managing psychiatric disorders, especially in complex cases involving comorbidities or polypharmacy. Pharmacist practitioners play a key role in optimizing medication regimens, educating patients, and ensuring adherence. Effective communication between healthcare providers, facilitated by structured tools and shared decision-making, improves patient outcomes and enhances the overall quality of psychiatric care. Case studies illustrate the practical benefits of interprofessional collaboration in delivering patient-centered, integrated care.

References:

1. American Psychiatric Association. (2016). **The Collaborative Care Model: An Approach for Integrating Physical and Mental Health Care in Medicaid Health Homes**.
2. Katon, W., Unützer, J., & Wells, K. (2010). Collaborative care models: An evidence-based approach to integrating physical and mental health care. *The Lancet*, 374(9690), 1211-1213.
3. Kovich, H., & Dejong, A. (2015). Integrating mental health and primary care. *American Family Physician*, 91(9), 647-652.
4. Rollman, B. L., Belnap, B. H., Mazumdar, S., et al. (2014). The efficacy of collaborative care for treating depression in older primary care patients: A randomized trial. *JAMA Internal Medicine*, 174(5), 776-785.
5. Unützer, J., Harbin, H., Schoenbaum, M., & Druss, B. (2013). The collaborative care model: An approach for integrating mental health care into primary care settings. *American Journal of Managed Care*, 19(5), 354-358.
6. Smith, R. C., Lein, C., Collins, C., et al. (2018). Treating patients with multiple chronic conditions: A case-based discussion. *Journal of Clinical Outcomes Management*, 25(3), 112-120.

Chapter 17: Ethical and Legal Considerations in Psychiatric Practice

Ethical and legal considerations play a central role in psychiatric practice, as mental health care often involves complex decisions about autonomy, informed consent, confidentiality, and the balance between patient rights and public safety. Mental health professionals must navigate these ethical and legal challenges while adhering to core ethical principles and professional responsibilities.

This chapter will explore the **ethical principles in mental health care delivery**, the **legal issues and regulations** governing psychiatric practice, key concepts such as **informed consent**, **confidentiality**, and **patient rights**, as well as the **ethical dilemmas** faced by pharmacist practitioners and other professionals in psychiatric care.

17.1. Ethical Principles in Mental Health Care Delivery

17.1.1. Autonomy:

The principle of autonomy emphasizes the right of patients to make decisions about their own health care based on **informed consent** and **self-determination**. In psychiatric practice, respecting autonomy can be challenging, particularly when a patient's mental health condition impairs their ability to make informed decisions.

- **Competence and Capacity**: Determining a patient's competence to make decisions is critical in psychiatric care. Competence refers to a patient's legal ability to make decisions, while **decision-making capacity** refers to their ability to understand information, weigh the risks and benefits, and communicate a choice.
- **Involuntary Treatment**: In some cases, patients with severe mental illness may lack decision-making capacity, raising ethical questions about involuntary treatment. While autonomy is a central ethical principle, it must be balanced with **beneficence** (acting in the patient's best interest) and **non-maleficence** (preventing harm).

17.1.2. Beneficence and Non-Maleficence:

- **Beneficence** refers to the obligation of healthcare providers to act in the best interest of the patient, promoting well-being and offering treatments that improve mental health outcomes.
- **Non-maleficence** means "do no harm." In psychiatric practice, this principle requires careful consideration when prescribing medications, performing procedures (e.g., electroconvulsive therapy), or recommending treatments that may have side effects or potential risks.

These principles often come into conflict, particularly in situations where a treatment may benefit a patient but also carries significant risks, such as the use of **antipsychotics** in elderly patients with dementia who may be at risk for cardiovascular complications.

17.1.3. Justice:

The principle of justice involves ensuring **fair and equitable access** to mental health care for all patients, regardless of their background, financial status, or geographic location. In mental health, this often includes addressing health disparities in underserved populations and ensuring that vulnerable groups (e.g., racial and ethnic minorities, individuals with disabilities) receive appropriate care.

- **Distributive Justice**: This concept focuses on the fair allocation of limited healthcare resources. In psychiatric care, this may involve decisions about **allocation of services** (e.g., access to inpatient care) or **funding** for mental health programs.

17.2. Legal Issues and Regulations Governing Psychiatric Practice

17.2.1. Mental Health Laws and Regulations:

Mental health care is subject to a range of legal frameworks that regulate the treatment of individuals with mental illness. These laws vary by jurisdiction but share common principles aimed at protecting patient rights while ensuring public safety.

- **Involuntary Commitment**: In cases where individuals pose a danger to themselves or others, mental health professionals may pursue involuntary commitment under civil commitment laws. The criteria for involuntary commitment typically include evidence of **imminent harm** and a lack of decision-making capacity.
- **Competency and Guardianship**: Patients who are unable to make informed decisions about their care may be deemed incompetent by a court. In such cases, a legal **guardian** may be appointed to make decisions on the patient's behalf.

17.2.2. HIPAA and Confidentiality:

The **Health Insurance Portability and Accountability Act (HIPAA)** establishes national standards for the protection of patient health information, including in psychiatric care. Confidentiality is a cornerstone of the patient-provider relationship, but there are exceptions in psychiatric practice that balance confidentiality with public safety.

- **Exceptions to Confidentiality**: Mental health professionals may be required to breach confidentiality in certain situations, such as when a patient poses a threat to others. The **Tarasoff ruling** established a legal duty to **warn potential victims** if a patient presents a credible threat of harm.

17.2.3. Informed Consent in Psychiatric Treatment:

Informed consent is a legal and ethical requirement in psychiatric practice, ensuring that patients understand the nature of their treatment, potential risks, and alternatives before agreeing to proceed.

- **Informed Consent Process**: For consent to be valid, the patient must be informed of their condition, the proposed treatment, possible side effects, and alternative options, and must voluntarily agree to treatment without coercion.
- **Challenges in Psychiatric Settings**: Obtaining informed consent in psychiatric practice can be complicated by conditions such as **psychosis, severe depression**, or **cognitive impairments** that may affect a patient's decision-making capacity. In these cases, a surrogate decision-maker may be needed, and treatment may require judicial review.

17.3. Informed Consent, Confidentiality, and Patient Rights in Psychiatric Treatment

17.3.1. Informed Consent:

As previously discussed, informed consent in psychiatric care is vital to respecting patient autonomy. However, in some cases, the patient may not fully understand their condition or treatment options due to mental health symptoms, creating an ethical dilemma for practitioners.

- **Emergency Situations**: In emergency situations where a patient is unable to consent and immediate treatment is necessary to prevent harm, treatment may proceed without formal consent. However, efforts to involve family members or legal representatives should be made whenever possible.

17.3.2. Confidentiality:

Maintaining patient confidentiality is essential for fostering trust in the therapeutic relationship. Psychiatric information, particularly related to diagnosis and treatment, is sensitive and requires careful handling.

- **Minors and Confidentiality**: Special challenges arise when treating minors, as confidentiality must be balanced with parental involvement. Generally, parents or guardians have the right to access a minor's medical records, but certain aspects of psychiatric care, such as discussions of sexual activity or substance use, may be protected depending on state laws.

17.3.3. Patient Rights:

Patients with mental health conditions have specific legal rights to ensure they receive appropriate care while protecting their autonomy and dignity.

- **Right to Refuse Treatment**: Patients generally have the right to refuse treatment, even in psychiatric settings. However, exceptions may occur if the patient lacks capacity or poses an immediate danger. In such cases, the decision to override patient refusal must be justified by clinical and legal standards.

- **Right to Access Records**: Under HIPAA, patients have the right to access their medical records, including psychiatric treatment records, unless this poses a substantial risk to their well-being. Providers may withhold certain sensitive information under these circumstances but must document the reasoning.

17.4. Ethical Dilemmas and Professional Responsibilities of Pharmacist Practitioners

Pharmacist practitioners in mental health care face unique ethical challenges, particularly in balancing patient safety with autonomy, addressing medication-related issues, and collaborating with other healthcare providers.

17.4.1. Balancing Autonomy and Safety in Medication Management:

Pharmacists have a duty to ensure that medications are prescribed appropriately, taking into account the patient's condition, treatment goals, and potential risks. However, ethical dilemmas can arise when a patient refuses medication or exhibits poor adherence to treatment.

- **Patient Refusal of Medication**: If a patient refuses to take prescribed psychotropic medications, the pharmacist must respect the patient's autonomy while also advocating for their well-being. This may involve exploring alternative treatments, educating the patient on the risks of non-adherence, or working with the healthcare team to adjust the treatment plan.
- **Polypharmacy and Deprescribing**: Pharmacists often encounter situations where a patient is prescribed multiple psychotropic medications (polypharmacy), which can lead to increased risk of adverse effects. Pharmacists have an ethical responsibility to **recommend deprescribing** or adjusting regimens to optimize safety and efficacy, particularly in vulnerable populations such as the elderly.

17.4.2. Conflicts of Interest:

Pharmacists may face conflicts of interest when there is pressure to prescribe certain medications due to institutional policies, financial incentives, or relationships with pharmaceutical companies. Pharmacists must prioritize the best interest of the patient and avoid any real or perceived conflicts of interest.

- **Transparency and Integrity**: Ethical practice requires transparency in decision-making and ensuring that all medication recommendations are based on evidence and patient needs, rather than external pressures.

17.4.3. Collaborating with Other Healthcare Providers:

Pharmacists in psychiatric care often collaborate with psychiatrists, primary care providers, nurses, and social workers to manage patient care. Ethical dilemmas may arise when there is disagreement about the best course of treatment.

- **Interprofessional Collaboration**: Pharmacists have a professional responsibility to advocate for the patient's safety and well-being, even if this involves challenging the treatment decisions of other healthcare providers. This should be done respectfully and in the context of open communication and shared decision-making.

Ethical and legal considerations in psychiatric practice are complex and multifaceted, involving key principles such as autonomy, beneficence, non-maleficence, and justice. Mental health professionals, including pharmacist practitioners, must navigate these principles while ensuring that patients' rights to informed consent, confidentiality, and fair treatment are respected.

Addressing ethical dilemmas, managing medication safety, and balancing patient autonomy with public safety are central to the ethical responsibilities of healthcare providers. A strong understanding of legal regulations and ethical frameworks is essential for providing high-quality, patient-centered psychiatric care.

References:

1. American Psychiatric Association. (2013). *The Principles of Medical Ethics with Annotations Especially Applicable to Psychiatry* (2013 ed.).
2. Beauchamp, T. L., & Childress, J. F. (2019). **Principles of Biomedical Ethics** (8th ed.). New York, NY: Oxford University Press.
3. Appelbaum, P. S. (2007). Assessment of patients' competence to consent to treatment. *New England Journal of Medicine*, 357(18), 1834-1840.
4. American Pharmacists Association. (2017). Code of Ethics for Pharmacists. Retrieved from https://www.pharmacist.com
5. Jonsen, A. R., Siegler, M., & Winslade, W. J. (2010). **Clinical Ethics: A Practical Approach to Ethical Decisions in Clinical Medicine** (7th ed.). New York, NY: McGraw-Hill Education.
6. Tarasoff v. Regents of the University of California, 17 Cal. 3d 425 (1976).
7. Gutheil, T. G., & Appelbaum, P. S. (2000). Clinical Handbook of Psychiatry and the Law (4th ed.). Baltimore, MD: Lippincott Williams & Wilkins.

Chapter 18: Future Directions in Psychiatric Pharmacotherapy

Psychiatric pharmacotherapy is evolving rapidly, with advances in neuroscience, genetics, and technology opening up new possibilities for treatment. Emerging trends in drug development, personalized medicine, and digital therapeutics are shaping the future of mental health care. Pharmacist practitioners play a crucial role in these advancements, helping to optimize medication management and integrate new therapies into clinical practice.

This chapter explores the **emerging trends and innovations** in psychiatric drug development, the rise of **personalized medicine, advancements in neurotechnology and digital therapeutics**, and the expanding **opportunities for advanced pharmacist practitioners** in this dynamic field.

18.1. Emerging Trends and Innovations in Psychiatric Drug Development

18.1.1. Novel Mechanisms of Action in Drug Development:

Traditional psychiatric medications, such as **antidepressants**, **antipsychotics**, and **anxiolytics**, largely target the monoaminergic systems (e.g., serotonin, dopamine, norepinephrine). However, many patients do not respond adequately to these treatments, prompting the development of drugs that work through novel mechanisms.

- **Glutamatergic Agents**: Research into the role of the **glutamatergic system** in mood regulation and cognition has led to the development of new treatments for conditions like depression and schizophrenia. **Esketamine** (Spravato), an NMDA receptor antagonist, represents a breakthrough in treating **treatment-resistant depression**, offering rapid antidepressant effects via modulation of glutamate pathways. Additional compounds targeting the glutamatergic system are in development, with potential applications in **bipolar disorder** and **schizophrenia**.
- **Psychedelic-Assisted Therapy**: Psychedelics such as **psilocybin** and **MDMA** (3,4-methylenedioxymethamphetamine) are being studied for their therapeutic potential in **post-traumatic stress disorder (PTSD), depression**, and **addiction**. Early clinical trials have demonstrated promising results, with MDMA-assisted therapy granted **breakthrough therapy** designation by the FDA for PTSD.
- **Neuroinflammation Modulators**: Increasing evidence suggests that **neuroinflammation** plays a role in psychiatric disorders like **depression**, **schizophrenia**, and **Alzheimer's disease**. Drugs targeting inflammatory pathways, such as **anti-cytokine therapies**, are being investigated for their potential to improve outcomes in patients whose symptoms are linked to inflammation.

18.1.2. Pioneering Treatments for Specific Psychiatric Conditions:

- **Rapid-Acting Antidepressants**: Traditional antidepressants (e.g., SSRIs, SNRIs) take weeks to achieve their full effects. In contrast, drugs like **esketamine** offer rapid relief, within hours, making them crucial for patients with **acute suicidal ideation** or **treatment-resistant depression**. These rapid-acting agents are opening new avenues for managing depression, particularly in emergency psychiatric settings.
- **Cannabinoid-Based Therapies**: Research into **cannabinoids** is expanding beyond pain management and epilepsy. **Cannabidiol (CBD)**, a non-psychoactive component of cannabis, is being explored for its potential to treat **anxiety**, **schizophrenia**, and other psychiatric disorders, with some studies suggesting it has anxiolytic and antipsychotic effects.

18.2. Personalized Medicine Approaches in Psychiatric Care

Advances in **personalized medicine** are transforming psychiatric care by offering a more tailored approach to treatment, focusing on an individual's unique genetic, biological, and clinical profile. Personalized medicine in psychiatry is helping clinicians improve outcomes by moving beyond the traditional "one-size-fits-all" approach and toward more targeted therapies that address the complexities of each patient's condition. Two key areas of innovation are **pharmacogenomics** and the use of **biomarkers** and **predictive analytics**.

18.2.1. Pharmacogenomics in Psychiatry

Pharmacogenomics is the study of how an individual's genetic makeup influences their response to medications. In psychiatry, where treatment responses can vary widely between patients, pharmacogenomics is playing an increasingly critical role in optimizing medication choices and dosages. This field is particularly important in mental health care, where **trial-and-error** prescribing can lead to delays in symptom relief, unwanted side effects, or treatment discontinuation.

CYP450 Enzymes and Drug Metabolism

A significant portion of pharmacogenomic research in psychiatry focuses on variations in the **cytochrome P450** (CYP450) enzyme family, particularly **CYP2D6** and **CYP2C19**, which are responsible for metabolizing many psychotropic medications, including **antidepressants**, **antipsychotics**, and **mood stabilizers**.

- **CYP2D6 Variations**:
    - **Poor metabolizers** of CYP2D6 may have elevated levels of medications like **fluoxetine** or **risperidone**, leading to an increased risk of side effects such as sedation, weight gain, or extrapyramidal symptoms.
    - **Ultrarapid metabolizers** may metabolize these drugs too quickly, resulting in subtherapeutic drug levels and insufficient symptom control.
- **CYP2C19 Variations**:
    - Variations in **CYP2C19** can affect the metabolism of **SSRIs** like **escitalopram** and **sertraline**, impacting efficacy and side effects. For example, poor

metabolizers of CYP2C19 may experience excessive drug accumulation, increasing the risk of side effects like sexual dysfunction or nausea.

Pharmacogenomic testing allows clinicians to identify these genetic variations, guiding medication selection and dosing to improve patient outcomes and reduce the risk of adverse effects.

Personalized Treatment Plans

Genetic testing can also help predict individual responses to psychiatric medications, allowing clinicians to develop more **personalized treatment plans**. For example:

- **SLC6A4 Gene**: Variations in the **SLC6A4** gene, which encodes the **serotonin transporter**, can influence how a patient responds to **Selective Serotonin Reuptake Inhibitors (SSRIs)**. Patients with certain variants may have a reduced response to SSRIs, helping clinicians consider alternative treatments, such as **serotonin-norepinephrine reuptake inhibitors (SNRIs)** or non-pharmacological therapies like **Cognitive Behavioral Therapy (CBT)** earlier in the treatment process.

By incorporating pharmacogenomics into clinical practice, providers can minimize the need for trial-and-error prescribing, resulting in faster relief of symptoms and fewer medication adjustments.

18.2.2. Biomarkers and Predictive Analytics

The identification of **biomarkers** and the use of **predictive analytics** are promising approaches for enhancing personalized medicine in psychiatry. These tools can help clinicians predict treatment responses, optimize treatment strategies, and provide more **targeted interventions** for psychiatric disorders.

Biomarkers for Depression

Biomarkers are biological indicators that can offer insights into the underlying mechanisms of psychiatric disorders and how patients are likely to respond to certain treatments. In depression, several potential biomarkers are being studied:

- **Inflammatory Markers**: Elevated levels of **C-reactive protein (CRP)** and other inflammatory markers have been associated with **treatment-resistant depression**. Identifying patients with high levels of inflammation may help guide treatment decisions, such as using anti-inflammatory agents or medications with anti-inflammatory properties (e.g., **ketamine** or **bupropion**).
- **Brain-Derived Neurotrophic Factor (BDNF)**: BDNF is a protein involved in **neuroplasticity** and is believed to play a role in the pathophysiology of depression. Low levels of BDNF have been linked to poor response to antidepressants. Monitoring BDNF levels could help predict which patients are likely to benefit from traditional **antidepressant therapy** versus those who may require alternative or adjunctive

treatments (e.g., **electroconvulsive therapy (ECT)** or **transcranial magnetic stimulation (TMS)**).
- **Cortisol Levels**: Dysregulated **cortisol** patterns, such as elevated morning cortisol, have been associated with depression and may help identify individuals who would benefit from treatments targeting the **hypothalamic-pituitary-adrenal (HPA)** axis.

By using biomarkers, clinicians can take a more **targeted approach** to treating depression, reducing the time spent on ineffective therapies and improving overall outcomes.

Predictive Analytics and Artificial Intelligence (AI)

The integration of **predictive analytics** and **artificial intelligence (AI)** in psychiatric care is helping clinicians make more **data-driven decisions**. AI and machine learning algorithms can analyze large sets of data, including **genetic information**, **clinical history**, and **biomarker levels**, to predict which treatments are most likely to succeed for an individual patient.

- **Example**: AI models are being developed to analyze patterns in **electronic health records (EHRs)** to predict **treatment outcomes** for patients with depression. These models can incorporate data on **prior medication responses**, **genetic factors**, and **lifestyle** (e.g., sleep patterns, activity levels) to suggest the most appropriate treatment plans.
- **Machine Learning in Schizophrenia**: Predictive analytics is also being used in **schizophrenia** care to identify patients at high risk of **relapse**. Machine learning models can analyze **medication adherence**, **psychosocial stressors**, and **clinical symptoms** to alert providers to patients who may need more intensive monitoring or intervention.

Predictive analytics tools are still in development, but they hold great promise in providing **personalized, data-driven treatment plans** for psychiatric patients, allowing for earlier intervention and more precise care.

18.3. Advancements in Neurotechnology and Digital Therapeutics

18.3.1. Neurostimulation Technologies:

Neurostimulation technologies are emerging as promising non-pharmacological treatments for psychiatric disorders. These techniques modulate brain activity to improve symptoms of conditions such as depression, anxiety, and PTSD.

- **Transcranial Magnetic Stimulation (TMS)**: TMS uses magnetic fields to stimulate specific brain regions, such as the **prefrontal cortex**, to alleviate symptoms of depression, particularly in patients who have not responded to medications. TMS is FDA-approved for **treatment-resistant depression** and is being studied for use in other conditions, including **OCD** and **bipolar disorder**.
- **Deep Brain Stimulation (DBS)**: DBS involves surgically implanting electrodes in specific brain regions to modulate neural activity. Initially used to treat movement

disorders like Parkinson's disease, DBS is now being explored for **treatment-resistant depression**, **obsessive-compulsive disorder**, and **Tourette syndrome**.
- **Vagus Nerve Stimulation (VNS)**: VNS, which stimulates the vagus nerve, has shown promise in treating **depression** and **epilepsy**. Researchers are also investigating its potential in treating **anxiety disorders** and **bipolar disorder**.

18.3.2. Digital Therapeutics and Mobile Health Technologies:

Digital therapeutics are software-based interventions designed to treat mental health conditions, often delivered via mobile apps or wearable devices.

- **Cognitive Behavioral Therapy (CBT) Apps**: Digital platforms offering **CBT** are increasingly used to treat depression, anxiety, and insomnia. Apps like **Woebot**, **Happify**, and **Headspace** provide evidence-based therapies that can be accessed anytime, improving access to mental health care, particularly in underserved populations.
- **Mobile Health for Symptom Monitoring**: Wearable devices and smartphone apps can monitor **sleep patterns**, **activity levels**, and **mood** in real-time, allowing for continuous symptom tracking. These tools can alert clinicians to early signs of relapse or deterioration in mental health, enabling more timely interventions.

18.3.3. Virtual Reality (VR) in Psychiatry:

Virtual reality is being explored as a treatment tool in psychiatric care, particularly for **anxiety disorders** and **PTSD**.

- **VR Exposure Therapy**: VR allows patients to safely engage in **exposure therapy** for conditions like **phobias**, **PTSD**, and **social anxiety disorder** by simulating feared environments in a controlled setting. This approach provides immersive, real-life scenarios that help patients confront and manage their fears gradually.
- **VR for Social Skills Training**: For individuals with **autism spectrum disorder (ASD)** or **schizophrenia**, VR can be used to simulate social interactions, helping patients practice social skills in a safe and supportive environment.

18.4. Opportunities for Advanced Pharmacist Practitioners in Advancing Psychiatric Pharmacotherapy

Pharmacist practitioners are uniquely positioned to play a key role in the future of psychiatric pharmacotherapy, particularly as new treatments and technologies become available.

18.4.1. Pharmacogenomic Testing and Personalized Medicine:

Pharmacists can lead efforts in **pharmacogenomic testing**, interpreting genetic results and recommending personalized medication regimens for patients based on their genetic profiles. By guiding clinicians in selecting the most appropriate medications, pharmacists help reduce the trial-and-error process, minimize side effects, and improve treatment outcomes.

- **Education and Implementation**: Pharmacists can educate both patients and healthcare providers about the benefits of pharmacogenomic testing, ensuring that it is integrated into routine psychiatric care.

18.4.2. Medication Management in Neurostimulation and Digital Therapeutics:

As **neurostimulation** and **digital therapeutics** become more integrated into psychiatric care, pharmacists will play an important role in managing medications alongside these new therapies.

- **Combination Therapy**: Pharmacists can optimize treatment regimens for patients receiving both psychotropic medications and neurostimulation therapies (e.g., TMS, DBS), ensuring there are no adverse interactions and that the overall treatment plan is effective.
- **Digital Therapeutic Monitoring**: Pharmacists can monitor patients using digital therapeutics, such as mobile health apps, ensuring that medication regimens are aligned with digital interventions to provide a comprehensive approach to mental health care.

18.4.3. Role in Clinical Trials and Research:

Pharmacists have the opportunity to contribute to **clinical trials** of new psychiatric medications, neurostimulation technologies, and digital therapeutics. Their expertise in medication management, pharmacodynamics, and patient care makes them valuable team members in research settings.

- **Investigational Drug Management**: Pharmacists can oversee the dispensing and monitoring of investigational drugs in clinical trials, ensuring that protocols are followed, and adverse effects are reported promptly.
- **Advancing Knowledge in Psychiatric Pharmacotherapy**: By participating in clinical research, pharmacists contribute to the growing body of knowledge in psychiatric pharmacotherapy, helping bring new and effective treatments to patients faster.

The future of psychiatric pharmacotherapy is shaped by innovations in drug development, personalized medicine, neurotechnology, and digital therapeutics. These advances offer exciting opportunities to improve the effectiveness and accessibility of mental health care. Pharmacist practitioners will play an increasingly important role in guiding the integration of these innovations into clinical practice, from pharmacogenomic testing and medication management to supporting the use of neurostimulation and digital health technologies. By staying at the forefront of these advancements, pharmacists can help ensure that psychiatric care is both personalized and cutting-edge, leading to better outcomes for patients with mental health conditions.

References:

1. Krystal, J. H., Sanacora, G., & Duman, R. S. (2019). Rapid-acting glutamatergic antidepressants: The path to ketamine and beyond. *Biological Psychiatry*, 85(6), 388-398.
2. Vollenweider, F. X., & Kometer, M. (2010). The neurobiology of psychedelic drugs: Implications for the treatment of mood disorders. *Nature Reviews Neuroscience*, 11(9), 642-651.
3. Warden, D., Rush, A. J., Trivedi, M. H., et al. (2007). The STAR*D project results: A comprehensive review of findings. *Current Psychiatry Reports*, 9(6), 449-459.
4. Egerton, A., & Stone, J. M. (2012). Glutamate and dopamine dysfunction in schizophrenia: An update. *Progress in Brain Research*, 211, 1-28.
5. Domschke, K., & Maron, E. (2013). Pharmacogenetics of anxiety disorders. *Pharmacology & Therapeutics*, 138(1), 37-52.
6. McGough, J. J., & Loo, S. K. (2014). Neurostimulation in pediatric psychiatry: TMS, tDCS, and ECT. *Journal of the American Academy of Child & Adolescent Psychiatry*, 53(12), 1299-1311.
7. Karyotaki, E., Ebert, D. D., Donkin, L., et al. (2018). Do guided internet-based interventions result in clinically relevant symptom reduction for adults with depressive symptoms? A meta-analysis of individual participant data. *JAMA Psychiatry*, 75(7), 711-719.

Chapter 19. Appendices

19.1. Commonly used psychiatric medications: dosing, indications, and adverse effects

19.2. Clinical assessment tools and screening instruments for psychiatric disorders

19.3. Resources for patients and caregivers: support groups, helplines, and educational materials

19.1. Appendix 1: Commonly Used Psychiatric Medications – Dosing, Indications, and Adverse Effects

This appendix provides an overview of commonly used psychiatric medications, including **antidepressants**, **antipsychotics**, **anxiolytics**, **mood stabilizers**, and **stimulants**. It covers their dosing, indications, and potential adverse effects to aid in clinical decision-making.

19.1.1. Antidepressants

Medication	Class	Indications	Typical Dosing	Common Adverse Effects
Fluoxetine (Prozac)	SSRI	Depression, anxiety, OCD	20-80 mg/day	Insomnia, sexual dysfunction, nausea
Sertraline (Zoloft)	SSRI	Depression, PTSD, anxiety	50-200 mg/day	GI upset, insomnia, sexual dysfunction
Venlafaxine (Effexor)	SNRI	Depression, GAD, panic disorder	75-225 mg/day	Hypertension, sweating, withdrawal symptoms
Bupropion (Wellbutrin)	NDRI	Depression, smoking cessation	150-450 mg/day	Insomnia, dry mouth, seizures (rare)

Medication	Class	Indications	Typical Dosing	Common Adverse Effects
Amitriptyline (Elavil)	TCA	Depression, neuropathic pain	25-150 mg/day	Sedation, weight gain, anticholinergic effects

19.1.2. Antipsychotics

Medication	Class	Indications	Typical Dosing	Common Adverse Effects
Risperidone (Risperdal)	Atypical Antipsychotic	Schizophrenia, bipolar disorder	1-6 mg/day	Weight gain, hyperprolactinemia, sedation
Quetiapine (Seroquel)	Atypical Antipsychotic	Schizophrenia, bipolar disorder	50-800 mg/day	Sedation, weight gain, orthostatic hypotension
Haloperidol (Haldol)	Typical Antipsychotic	Schizophrenia, acute agitation	1-10 mg/day	Extrapyramidal symptoms (EPS), tardive dyskinesia
Aripiprazole (Abilify)	Atypical Antipsychotic	Schizophrenia, bipolar disorder	10-30 mg/day	Akathisia, GI upset, insomnia
Clozapine (Clozaril)	Atypical Antipsychotic	Treatment-resistant schizophrenia	300-900 mg/day	Agranulocytosis, weight gain, sedation

19.1.3. Anxiolytics

Medication	Class	Indications	Typical Dosing	Common Adverse Effects
Lorazepam (Ativan)	Benzodiazepine	Anxiety, acute agitation, status epilepticus	0.5-4 mg/day	Sedation, dependence, withdrawal
Buspirone (Buspar)	Non-benzodiazepine anxiolytic	Generalized anxiety disorder (GAD)	15-60 mg/day	Dizziness, nausea, headaches
Clonazepam (Klonopin)	Benzodiazepine	Panic disorder, seizure disorders	0.5-4 mg/day	Sedation, cognitive impairment, tolerance

19.1.4. Mood Stabilizers

Medication	Class	Indications	Typical Dosing	Common Adverse Effects
Lithium (Lithobid)	Mood Stabilizer	Bipolar disorder (mania, maintenance)	300-1800 mg/day	Tremor, weight gain, hypothyroidism, renal impairment
Valproate (Depakote)	Anticonvulsant	Bipolar disorder, seizure disorders	750-1500 mg/day	GI upset, weight gain, liver toxicity

Medication	Class	Indications	Typical Dosing	Common Adverse Effects
Lamotrigine (Lamictal)	Anticonvulsant	Bipolar depression, seizure disorders	100-400 mg/day	Rash (risk of Stevens-Johnson syndrome), headaches

19.1.5. Stimulants

Medication	Class	Indications	Typical Dosing	Common Adverse Effects
Methylphenidate (Ritalin)	Stimulant	ADHD, narcolepsy	10-60 mg/day	Insomnia, decreased appetite, irritability
Amphetamine (Adderall)	Stimulant	ADHD, narcolepsy	5-40 mg/day	Insomnia, weight loss, increased heart rate

19.2. Appendix 2: Clinical Assessment Tools and Screening Instruments for Psychiatric Disorders

19.2.1. Depression

- **Patient Health Questionnaire-9 (PHQ-9)**: A 9-item screening tool for depression that evaluates the severity of depressive symptoms and monitors response to treatment. A score of 10 or higher suggests moderate depression, requiring further evaluation.
- **Beck Depression Inventory (BDI)**: A widely used 21-item self-report questionnaire assessing the severity of depression.

19.2.2. Anxiety

- **Generalized Anxiety Disorder-7 (GAD-7)**: A 7-item questionnaire that screens for generalized anxiety disorder and assesses the severity of symptoms. Scores of 5, 10, and 15 represent mild, moderate, and severe anxiety, respectively.
- **Hamilton Anxiety Rating Scale (HAM-A)**: A clinician-administered scale that measures the severity of anxiety symptoms in 14 categories, including somatic complaints and mood-related symptoms.

19.2.3. Bipolar Disorder

- **Mood Disorder Questionnaire (MDQ)**: A screening tool for bipolar disorder that assesses the presence of manic or hypomanic episodes. A positive score indicates the need for further diagnostic evaluation.

19.2.4. Substance Use Disorders

- **Alcohol Use Disorders Identification Test (AUDIT)**: A 10-item screening tool developed by the World Health Organization to assess harmful alcohol use. A score of 8 or more indicates hazardous or harmful alcohol consumption.
- **CAGE Questionnaire**: A brief 4-question screening tool for alcohol use disorder, focusing on **C**utting down, **A**nnoyance by criticism, **G**uilt about drinking, and **E**ye-openers.

19.2.5. Psychosis

- **Positive and Negative Syndrome Scale (PANSS)**: A clinician-administered tool used to assess the severity of positive and negative symptoms in schizophrenia, including hallucinations, delusions, and social withdrawal.

19.2.6. Cognitive Impairment

- **Mini-Mental State Examination (MMSE)**: A widely used 30-point test that measures cognitive impairment in patients with suspected dementia or other neurocognitive disorders. Scores below 24 indicate cognitive impairment.
- **Montreal Cognitive Assessment (MoCA)**: A more sensitive tool than the MMSE for detecting mild cognitive impairment, with a total score of 30 points. Scores below 26 suggest cognitive impairment.

19.3. Appendix 3: Resources for Patients and Caregivers – Support Groups, Helplines, and Educational Materials

19.3.1. National and International Organizations

- **National Alliance on Mental Illness (NAMI)**: Offers free support groups, educational programs, and advocacy for individuals living with mental illness and their families. Website: www.nami.org
- **Mental Health America (MHA)**: Provides mental health screening tools, educational materials, and resources to promote mental wellness. Website: www.mhanational.org

19.3.2. Helplines

- **National Suicide Prevention Lifeline (USA)**: 1-800-273-TALK (8255). A 24/7 helpline for individuals in distress, providing free, confidential support and crisis intervention.
- **Crisis Text Line**: Text HOME to 741741 to connect with a crisis counselor in the U.S. or Canada, available 24/7 for support during emotional distress.

19.3.3. Support Groups

- **Depression and Bipolar Support Alliance (DBSA)**: Offers peer-led support groups for individuals living with mood disorders and their families. Website: www.dbsalliance.org
- **Alcoholics Anonymous (AA)**: A fellowship offering peer support for individuals recovering from alcohol addiction, based on a 12-step program. Website: www.aa.org
- **Narcotics Anonymous (NA)**: A global organization providing support for individuals recovering from drug addiction through peer-led groups. Website: www.na.org

19.3.4. Educational Materials and Online Resources

- **Mayo Clinic Psychiatry and Psychology Resources**: Provides reliable information on mental health conditions, treatments, and coping strategies. Website: www.mayoclinic.org
- **American Psychiatric Association (APA)**: Offers comprehensive guides and FAQs on various psychiatric disorders, including educational resources for patients and caregivers. Website: www.psychiatry.org
- **Child Mind Institute**: Provides educational content and resources for parents and caregivers of children with psychiatric disorders, including ADHD, anxiety, and depression. Website: www.childmind.org

---

These appendices offer practical information on psychiatric medications, clinical assessment tools, and resources for both healthcare providers and patients.

Chapter 20. Glossary: A-Z Definitions of key terms and concepts related to psychiatric disorders and pharmacotherapy

A

- **Affect**: The observable expression of emotion, often categorized as **blunted**, **flat**, **inappropriate**, or **labile**, depending on the intensity and appropriateness of emotional expression.
- **Akathisia**: A state of inner restlessness and inability to sit still, often a side effect of antipsychotic medications.
- **Anhedonia**: The inability to experience pleasure in activities that typically bring joy, a core symptom of depression.
- **Antidepressants**: A class of medications used to treat depressive disorders, anxiety disorders, and other mood-related conditions. Includes **SSRIs**, **SNRIs**, **TCAs**, and **MAOIs**.
- **Antipsychotics**: Medications used to manage psychotic disorders, including schizophrenia and bipolar disorder. Classified into **typical (first-generation)** and **atypical (second-generation)** antipsychotics.
- **Anxiolytics**: Medications that reduce anxiety, such as **benzodiazepines** and **non-benzodiazepine anxiolytics** (e.g., buspirone).

B

- **Benzodiazepines**: A class of anxiolytic medications used to treat anxiety, insomnia, and seizures. They work by enhancing the effect of **GABA** and include drugs like **lorazepam** and **diazepam**.
- **Bipolar Disorder**: A mood disorder characterized by alternating periods of **mania**, **hypomania**, and **depression**.
- **Black Box Warning**: The strictest warning issued by the FDA, indicating that a medication carries a significant risk of serious or life-threatening adverse effects.

C

- **Cognitive Behavioral Therapy (CBT)**: A structured form of psychotherapy that aims to modify dysfunctional thoughts and behaviors associated with various psychiatric disorders, particularly anxiety and depression.
- **Cognitive Impairment**: Difficulty with cognitive functions such as memory, attention, language, and executive functioning, commonly seen in disorders like dementia and schizophrenia.
- **Compliance/Adherence**: The extent to which a patient follows prescribed medication or therapy regimens. Non-adherence is a major challenge in psychiatric care.

- **Comorbidity**: The presence of one or more additional diseases or disorders co-occurring with a primary condition, such as **depression** and **anxiety** or **substance use disorder** with **schizophrenia**.

D

- **Delusions**: Fixed, false beliefs that are not aligned with reality and are resistant to reasoning or contrary evidence, commonly seen in **schizophrenia** and other psychotic disorders.
- **Depersonalization**: A feeling of being detached from one's own body or mental processes, as if observing oneself from outside.
- **Dopamine**: A neurotransmitter involved in regulating mood, cognition, and motor function. Dopamine dysregulation is implicated in conditions such as schizophrenia and Parkinson's disease.
- **DSM-5 (Diagnostic and Statistical Manual of Mental Disorders, Fifth Edition)**: The standard classification of mental disorders used by mental health professionals for diagnostic purposes.

E

- **Electroconvulsive Therapy (ECT)**: A medical treatment involving the application of electrical currents to the brain, used primarily for severe depression, bipolar disorder, and treatment-resistant schizophrenia.
- **Extrapyramidal Symptoms (EPS)**: Drug-induced movement disorders, including **tardive dyskinesia, akathisia, dystonia,** and **parkinsonism**, often associated with antipsychotic medications.

F

- **Flat Affect**: A severe reduction in emotional expressiveness, often seen in individuals with schizophrenia.
- **Functional Impairment**: A reduction in an individual's ability to perform everyday activities due to mental health symptoms, such as work, social, or self-care tasks.

G

- **GABA (Gamma-Aminobutyric Acid)**: The primary inhibitory neurotransmitter in the central nervous system, involved in reducing neuronal excitability. Medications like **benzodiazepines** and **barbiturates** enhance GABA activity to reduce anxiety.
- **Generalized Anxiety Disorder (GAD)**: A condition characterized by chronic, excessive worry about various aspects of life, accompanied by physical symptoms such as muscle tension and sleep disturbances.

H

- **Hallucinations**: Sensory perceptions that occur in the absence of an external stimulus, such as hearing voices or seeing things that are not there. Commonly seen in psychotic disorders.
- **Hypomania**: A milder form of **mania** characterized by elevated mood, increased activity or energy, but without the severe functional impairment seen in full manic episodes.

I

- **Insomnia**: Difficulty falling asleep, staying asleep, or waking too early, leading to daytime impairment. It can be a symptom of several psychiatric disorders, including depression and anxiety.
- **Involuntary Commitment**: The legal process by which an individual with severe mental illness is hospitalized against their will, typically when they pose a danger to themselves or others.

L

- **Lithium**: A mood stabilizer used primarily in the treatment of **bipolar disorder**, particularly for controlling manic episodes and reducing the risk of suicide.

M

- **Mania**: An elevated, expansive, or irritable mood lasting for at least one week, accompanied by increased energy, decreased need for sleep, and impulsive or risky behaviors. A hallmark of **bipolar I disorder**.
- **Monoamine Oxidase Inhibitors (MAOIs)**: A class of antidepressants that inhibit the breakdown of monoamines (serotonin, norepinephrine, dopamine) and are typically used in treatment-resistant depression. MAOIs require dietary restrictions to avoid hypertensive crises.
- **Mood Stabilizers**: Medications used to treat mood disorders, particularly **bipolar disorder**. They include **lithium**, **valproate**, and **lamotrigine**.

N

- **Neuroleptic Malignant Syndrome (NMS)**: A rare but potentially life-threatening reaction to antipsychotic medications, characterized by fever, muscle rigidity, altered mental status, and autonomic dysfunction.
- **Neurotransmitter**: A chemical messenger that transmits signals across synapses between neurons in the brain. Examples include **serotonin**, **dopamine**, and **norepinephrine**.

O

- **Obsessive-Compulsive Disorder (OCD)**: A disorder characterized by intrusive, unwanted thoughts (obsessions) and repetitive behaviors or mental acts (compulsions) performed to reduce distress.
- **Orexin**: A neurotransmitter involved in regulating wakefulness and arousal, with some medications targeting orexin receptors to treat **insomnia**.

P

- **Panic Disorder**: A condition marked by recurrent, unexpected **panic attacks**, which are sudden periods of intense fear or discomfort accompanied by physical symptoms such as heart palpitations, sweating, and shortness of breath.
- **Paranoia**: Irrational and persistent feelings of mistrust or suspicion, commonly seen in psychotic disorders like schizophrenia and in paranoid personality disorder.
- **Positive Symptoms**: Symptoms of schizophrenia that involve the presence of abnormal experiences, such as **hallucinations**, **delusions**, and **disorganized thinking**.

R

- **Rapid Cycling**: A form of **bipolar disorder** in which the individual experiences four or more mood episodes (mania, hypomania, or depression) within a year.
- **Reuptake Inhibitors**: Medications that block the reabsorption of neurotransmitters (e.g., serotonin, norepinephrine) into neurons, increasing their availability in the synaptic cleft. **SSRIs** and **SNRIs** are examples.

S

- **Selective Serotonin Reuptake Inhibitors (SSRIs)**: A class of antidepressants that increase serotonin levels in the brain by inhibiting its reuptake. Commonly used to treat depression, anxiety, and OCD.
- **Serotonin Syndrome**: A potentially life-threatening condition caused by excessive serotonin activity, typically due to drug interactions or overdose. Symptoms include agitation, confusion, rapid heart rate, and hyperthermia.
- **Stimulants**: Medications such as **methylphenidate** and **amphetamine** used to treat ADHD and narcolepsy by increasing dopamine and norepinephrine activity in the brain.

T

- **Tardive Dyskinesia (TD)**: A movement disorder caused by long-term use of antipsychotic medications, characterized by involuntary, repetitive movements, often of the face, tongue, and limbs.
- **Tricyclic Antidepressants (TCAs)**: An older class of antidepressants that block the reuptake of serotonin and norepinephrine, used less frequently due to their side effects, such as anticholinergic symptoms and cardiotoxicity.

V

- **Vagus Nerve Stimulation (VNS)**: A neuromodulation treatment that uses electrical impulses delivered to the vagus nerve to treat conditions such as **treatment-resistant depression** and **epilepsy**.

W

- **Withdrawal Syndrome**: A set of symptoms that occur when a person discontinues or reduces the use of a medication or substance to which they have developed dependence, such as **benzodiazepines** or **antidepressants**.

Z

- **Z-Drugs**: A class of non-benzodiazepine hypnotics (e.g., **zolpidem**, **eszopiclone**) used to treat insomnia by enhancing the activity of GABA receptors without the high risk of dependence associated with benzodiazepines.

This glossary provides a quick reference to key terms and concepts used in psychiatric practice and pharmacotherapy, offering foundational knowledge for healthcare providers working in the mental health field.

www.ingramcontent.com/pod-product-compliance
Lightning Source LLC
LaVergne TN
LVHW072125060526
838201LV00071B/4977